OXFORD MEDICAL PUBLICATIONS

Adult Congenital
Heart Disease

Oxford Specialist Handbooks in Cardiology

Adult Congenital Heart Disease

EDITED BY

Sara Thorne

Consultant Cardiologist,
University Hospitals Birmingham,
Birmingham, UK

Paul Clift

Consultant Cardiologist,
University Hospitals Birmingham,
Birmingham, UK

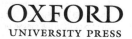

OXFORD
UNIVERSITY PRESS

OXFORD
UNIVERSITY PRESS

Great Clarendon Street, Oxford OX2 6DP

Oxford University Press is a department of the University of Oxford.
It furthers the University's objective of excellence in research, scholarship,
and education by publishing worldwide in

Oxford New York

Auckland Cape Town Dar es Salaam Hong Kong Karachi
Kuala Lumpur Madrid Melbourne Mexico City Nairobi
New Delhi Shanghai Taipei Toronto

With offices in

Argentina Austria Brazil Chile Czech Republic France Greece
Guatemala Hungary Italy Japan Poland Portugal Singapore
South Korea Switzerland Thailand Turkey Ukraine Vietnam

Oxford is a registered trade mark of Oxford University Press
in the UK and in certain other countries

Published in the United States
by Oxford University Press Inc., New York

British Library Cataloguing in Publication Data
Data available

Library of Congress Cataloging-in-Publication-Data
Data available

Typeset by Cepha Imaging Private Ltd., Bangalore, India
Printed in Italy
on acid-free paper by
L.E.G.O. S.p.A—Lavis TN

ISBN 978–0–19–922818–8

10 9 8 7 6 5 4 3 2 1

Foreword

This first edition of the *Adult Congenital Heart Disease* (part of the Oxford Specialist Handbooks in Cardiology series) fills an important void in the current letter literature about this topic. The authors intend to equip cardiology trainees, general cardiologists, and acute medicine physicians with a sound understanding of the principles of the physiology and management of adult congenital heart disease, so that they can treat emergencies and recognize the need for referral to a specialist unit. This book joins a large number of others in the Oxford Specialist Handbook series, in this case providing a practical approach to the investigation and treatment of adult patients with congenital heart defects.

Dr Sara Thorne and Dr Paul Clift, edited the entire text, giving this a consistent style and clinical approach that is welcome. Their style is to make simple clear assertions. The reader is treated to wonderfully straightforward recommendations that avoid needless complexities in the typical patient scenarios. The brevity of the text sometimes leaves the reader hoping to ask one of the authors to clarify their guidance. Information is presented in discrete chapters with a practical focus. Material is presented in point form or in brief sentences. The text is intended to remind the reader of things to check on things to do. The illustrations are very nicely labeled and reinforce what the clinician may be seeing in their own emergency department. There are very clear brief chapters on diagnostic methods and when/how to use them.

The diagnostic chapters are followed up by nine chapters on specific lesions in ACHD patients. These chapters deal with the main clinical issues that the reader may be encountering. Physical examination findings are nicely dealt with to support the clinician who only occasionally sees these types of patients.

There are other textbooks on adult congenital heart defects, but they are intended for medical personnel with an ongoing interest in and practice of adult congenital heart disease patients. The style of this handbook is reminiscent to me of the Canadian ACHD guidelines in their determination to be user friendly for the nonexpert in ACHD care in need of some guidance on a specific patient. The authors are to be congratulated for carrying off this challenge in such an admirable and readable way. Their book will be well received by clinicians who occasionally encounter ACHD patients, and who needs some straightforward advice as to how to go about competently managing the challenge.

Gary Webb, MD
Director
Philadelphia Adult Congenital Heart Center
Hospital of the University of Pennsylvania
Children's Hospital of Philadelphia,
Philadelphia, USA

Acknowledgements

We thank our patients for giving us the privilege of caring for them and discovering with them what their futures hold. We thank our many colleagues who together make up the adult congenital heart disease team. Lastly we thank our families for their continuing support and for helping us to keep it all in perspective.

Sara Thorne
Paul Clift

Contents

Introduction

The population of adults with congenital heart disease (ACHD, or GUCH; grown-up congenital heart disease) now exceeds that of children, and will continue to grow for at least the next 3 decades. Adult survivors have increasingly complex, surgically altered physiology and anatomy, and when complications occur, they can decompensate very quickly. The highly abnormal pathophysiology makes many patients particularly vulnerable to iatrogenic complications.

To the adult cardiologist, the language of congenital heart disease can be confusing and the spectrum of disease bewildering. Many find the prospect of meeting an adult with complex congenital heart disease in the emergency department disturbing, and rightly so.

This book aims to dispel confusion and equip cardiology trainees, general cardiologists, and acute medicine physicians with a sound understanding of the principles of the physiology and management of adult congenital heart disease, so that they can treat emergencies and recognize the need for referral to a specialist unit.

In the UK, clear guidance exists for the optimum structure of care for adults with congenital heart disease. A hub and spoke model is recommended, with 2-way communication between specialist centres, local hospitals, and other agencies (Fig. 1).

We hope that this book will provide a rapid reference with easy to understand diagrams and key clinical points, to look up when the clinical need arises. It also provides insight into the basic principles of congenital heart disease and should give the reader a good grounding in the care of the adult with congenital heart disease.

Further reading

Department of Health (2006). *Adult congenital heart disease. A commissioning guide for services for young people and grown ups with congenital heart disease (GUCH)*. Department of Health: London. ☙ www.dh.gov/publications

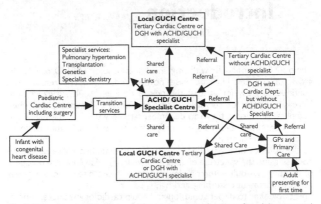

Fig. 1 Department of Health model for organization of services for adult congenital heart disease. ACHD adult congenital heart disease; DGH district general hospital; GUCH grown up congenital heart disease.

Contributors

David Barron
Consultant in Congenital Cardiac Surgery
Birmingham Children's Hospital Birmingham, UK
(Chapter 14)

Sarah Bowater
Cardiology SpR
University Hospitals Birmingham
Birmingham, UK
(Chapters 7, 11, 14, 16, Appendices)

Paul Clift (editor)
(Chapters 3, 4, 14)
Consultant Cardiologist
University Hospitals Birmingham
Birmingham, UK

Asle Hirth
Consultant Paediatric Cardiologist
Department of Heart Disease
Haukeland University Hospital
Bergen, Norway
(Chapters 3, 10, 12, 15, 19)

Lucy Hudsmith
Cardiology SpR
University Hospitals Birmingham,
Birmingham, UK
(Chapters 2, 8, 16, 17)

Sara Thorne (editor)
(Chapters 1, 6, 13, 17)
Consultant Cardiologist,
University Hospitals Birmingham,
Birmingham, UK

Symbols and abbreviations

📖	cross reference
↑	increased
↓	decreased
→	leading to
♂	male
♀	female
+ve	positive
−ve	negative
2D	2-dimensional
3D	3-dimensional
AA	ascending aorta
ACEI	angiotensin converting enzyme inhibitor
ACHD	adult congenital heart disease
AD	autosomal dominant
AP	aortopulmonary
AR	aortic regurgitation *or* autosomal recessive
AS	aortic stenosis
ASD	atrial septal defect
AT	anaerobic threshold
AV	atrioventricular
AoV	aortic valve
AVSD	atrioventricular septal defect
AVVR	atrioventricular valve regurgitation
bpm	beats per minute
BT	Blalock–Taussig
ccTGA	congenitally corrected transposition of the great arteries
CMR	cardiovascular magnetic resonance imaging
CO	cardiac output
CoA	coarctation of aorta
COC	combined oral contraceptive
CPEX	cardiopulmonary exercise testing
CS	coronary sinus
CT	computed tomography
CTR	cardiothoracic ratio
CVA	cerebrovascular accident
Cx	circumflex

CXR	chest X-ray
DA	descending aorta
DORV	double outlet right ventricle
DVT	deep vein thrombosis
ECG	electrocardiogram
EF	ejection fraction
FA	femoral artery
Fe	iron
FBC	full blood count
GA	general anaesthetic
GI	gastrointestinal
GU	genitourinary
Hct	haematocrit
HDU	high-dependency unit
HLHS	hypoplastic left heart syndrome
HR	heart rate
IART	intra-atrial reentrant tachycardia
im	intramuscular
INR	international normalized ratio
IUD	intrauterine device
IUS	intrauterine system
iv	intravenous
IVC	inferior vena cava
JVP	jugular venous pressure
L	left
LA	left atrium
LAD	left anterior descending
LAO	left anterior oblique
LFT	liver function test
LIMA	left internal mammary artery
LMS	left main stem
LPA	left pulmonary artery
LV	left ventricle
LVH	left ventricular hypertrophy
LVOT	left ventricular outflow tract
MAPCA	major aortopulmonary collateral arteries
MAPSE	mitral annular planar systolic excursion
mLA	mean left atrial pressure
MPA	main pulmonary artery
mPAP	mean pulmonary artery pressure

mRA	mean right atrial pressure
ms	millisecond
MS	mitral stenosis
MV	mitral valve
mVSD	muscular ventricular septal defect
NBM	nil by mouth
NSAIA	non-steroidal anti-inflammatory agent
P–A	posterior–anterior
PA	pulmonary artery
PAPVD	partial anomalous pulmonary venous drainage
PDA	patent ductus arteriosus
PFO	patent foramen ovale
PHT	pulmonary hypertension
PLE	protein-losing enteropathy
PR	pulmonary regurgitation
PS	pulmonary stenosis
PV	pulmonary vein
PVA	pulmonary venous atrium
pmVSD	perimembranous ventricular septal defect
R	right
RA	right atrium
RAO	right anterior oblique
RBBB	right bundle branch block
RCA	right coronary artery
RER	respiratory exchange ratio
RPA	right pulmonary artery
RV	right ventricle
RVH	right ventricular hypertrophy
SC	subcutaneous
SpR	specialist registrar
SR	sinus rhythm
SVA	systemic venous atrium
SVC	superior vena cava
SVR	systemic vascular resistance
TAPSE	tricuspid annular planar systolic excursion
TAPVD	total anomalous pulmonary venous drainage
TCPC	total cavopulmonary connection
TGA	transposition of the great arteries
TFT	thyroid function test
TLC	total lung capacity

TOE	tranoesophageal echocardiogram/echocardiography
TPG	transpulmonary gradient
TR	tricuspid regurgitation
TTE	transthoracic echocardiogram/echocardiography
TV	tricuspid valve
U&E	urea and electrolyte
VA	ventriculo-arterial
VC	vital capacity
VSD	ventricular septal defect

Detailed contents

Part 1

Introduction to adult congenital heart disease

Morphology and classification

Introduction

The classification and description of complex congenital heart disease is important to the understanding of the anatomy and physiology of the conditions.[1,2] It can appear intimidating; an overview to a rational approach is described here.

Physiological classification

📖 See Table 1.1.
- A condition may be acyanotic or cyanotic.
- Acyanotic conditions may have:
  - No shunt (i.e. no communication between the pulmonary and systemic circulations);

or
  - A left (L)-to-right (R) shunt.
- Cyanotic conditions all have a R-to-L shunt.
- The behaviour of a cyanotic lesion depends on whether pulmonary blood flow is high or low (📖 see p. 65, Chapter 7).

1 Ho SY, Baker EJ, Rigby ML, Anderson RH (1995). *Colour atlas of congenital heart disease. Morphological and clinical correlations.* Times Mirror Publications Mosby-Wolfe, London.

2 Anderson RH, Becker AE (1997). *Controversies in the description of congenitally malformed hearts.* Imperial College Press, London.

Table 1.1 Physiological Classification of Congenital Heart Disease

| | Acyanotic | | | Cyanotic—Obligatory right to left shunt | | | | | |
| | No shunt | Left to right shunt | | Eisenmenger syndrome | | High pulmonary blood flow | | Normal or low pulmonary blood flow | |
Level of lesion	Example of specific lesion	Level of shunt	Example of specific lesion	Level of shunt	Example of specific lesion	Level of shunt	Example of specific lesion	Level of shunt	Example of specific lesion
RV inflow	Ebstein's anomaly	Atrium	PAPVD ASD AVSD	Atrium	ASD AVSD	Atrial	Large ASD	Atrial, with obstruction to pulmonary blood flow	Severe PS with ASD, Left SVC to LA connection
LV inflow	Congenital MS, Cor triatriatum	Ventricle	VSD	Ventricle	VSD	Ventricular		Ventricular, with obstruction to pulmonary blood flow	Fallot, Pulmonary atresia VSD, Univentricular heart with PS
RV outflow	Infundibular stenosis, PS	Artery	PDA AP window	Artery	PDA	Arterial		Extra cardiac	Pulmonary AVM
LV outflow	Subaortic stenosis, Bicuspid AoV	Multiple	AVSD	Multiple	AVSD	Multiple			
Arterial	Supravalvar stenosis, CoA								

AP aortopulmonary, ASD atrial septal defect, AoV aortic valve, AVSD atrioventricular septal defect, CoA coarctation of aorta, LA left atrium, LV left ventricle, MS mitral stenosis, PAPVD partial anomalous pulmonary venous drainage, PDA patent ductus arteriosus, PS pulmonary stenosis, RV right ventricle, SVC superior vena cava, VSD ventricular septal defect

Sequential segmental analysis

Any heart can be described using this approach. Especially useful for complex lesions.

The heart has 3 segments:
- Atrial chambers.
- Ventricular mass.
- Great arteries.

Each segment and its connection to the next segment is described in turn:
- Arrangement of the atria (situs)—📖 see Atrial arrangement, p.8.
- Atrio-ventricular (AV) connections and the morphology of the AV valves:
  - *AV concordance* = normal; RA connects to RV via a tricuspid valve (TV), LA connects to LV via a mitral valve (MV).
  - *AV discordance* = abnormal; RA connects to LV via a MV; LA connects to the RV via a tvTV.
- Ventriculoarterial (VA) connections and the morphology of the great arteries:
  - *VA concordance* = normal; RV connects to PA via a pulmonary valve (PV), LV connects to aorta via an aortic valve.
  - *VA discordance* = abnormal; RV connects to aorta via and aortic valve, LV connects to PA via a PV.
- Associated malformations.

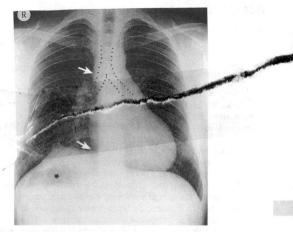

Fig. 1.1 Chest radiograph of a 50-year-old ♂ with abdominal situs inversus and laevocardia (*). Left atrial isomerism is inferred from the symmetrical long bronchi. The IVC is absent at the level of the diaphragm (small arrow) and the azygous vein receiving inferior caval venous blood is prominent (large arrow). Reproduced from Warrell D, Cox TM, Firth JM, *et al.* (eds) (2003). *Oxford Textbook of Medicine* 4th edn, p.1084, with permission from Oxford University Press.

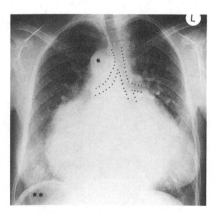

Fig. 1.2 Chest radiograph of a 21-year-old ♀ with abdominal situs inversus (**), bronchial and inferred atrial situs inversus, mesocardia, and right aortic arch (*). She has tetralogy of Fallot with pulmonary atresia with an aortopulmonary shunt via a left thoracotomy. Reproduced from Warrell D, Cox TM, Firth JM, *et al.* (eds) (2003). *Oxford Textbook of Medicine* 4th edn, p.1086, with permission from Oxford University Press.

Atrial arrangement

📖 See Table 1.2.
- Situs solitus: normal = usual arrangement of paired asymmetrical structures, i.e.:
  - Morphologic left atrium (LA) on the left and right atrium (RA) on the right.
  - Morphological left main bronchus on the left and right main bronchus on the right.
  - Stomach on the left, liver on the right.
- Situs inversus = mirror image arrangement of these structures.
- Isomerizm = abnormal symmetry of these structures.
  - Usually associated with coexistent complex lesions:
    —abnormal venous connections → technical difficulties at cardiac catheterization and permanent pacemaker insertion.
  - *Right isomerizm* more common in ♂. Survival to adulthood uncommon because of associated asplenia and severe cyanotic heart disease, including obstructed anomalous pulmonary venous drainage (the pulmonary venous confluence is a left atrial structure).
  - *Left isomerizm*: more common in ♀ associated lesions tend to produce L-to-R shunts and little if any cyanosis. Better prognosis than right isomerizm. In left isomerizm, there is usually interruption of the inferior vena cava (IVC), and the abdominal venous return connects to the heart via a (R-sided) azygos or (L-sided) hemiazygos vein. The hepatic veins can be identified draining separately into the atria.

Table 1.2 Atrial arrangement

	Atrial situs solitus: Normal	Atrial situs inversus	Right isomerizm	Left isomerizm
Atrial morphology	R-sided morphologic RA, L-sided morphologic LA.	Mirror image: R-sided morphologic LA, L-sided morphologic RA	Bilateral morphological RA.	Bilateral morphological LA.
Atrial appendages	Broad based RA appendage, long narrow LA appendage	Mirror image	Bilateral RA appendages	Bilateral LA appendages
Sinus node	Single, R-sided	Single, L-sided	Bilateral	Absent
Pulmonary morphology	R lung trilobed L lung bilobed	R lung bilobed L lung trilobed	Bilateral trilobed lungs	Bilateral Bilobed lungs
Bronchial morphology*	Short R-sided main bronchus, Long L- sided main bronchus:	Mirror image	Bilateral short morphological R bronchi	Bilateral long morphological L bronchi
Abdominal arrangement**				
Aorta & IVC	Aorta to L of spine, IVC to R of spine	Normal or mirror image	Aorta and IVC on same side. IVC anterior to aorta.	Aorta and azygos on same side. Azygos posterior to aorta.
Stomach	L-sided	Normal or mirror image	Usually L sided	Usually R sided
Liver	R-sided		Midline	Midline
Spleen	R-sided		Usually absent	Often polysplenia.

IVC, inferior vena cava; L, left; LA, left atrium; R, right; RA, right atrium; SVC, superior vena cava

*Since bronchopulmonary situs nearly always follows atrial situs, atrial situs can be inferred from the chest radiograph

**Echocardiography shows the intra-abdominal relations of the great vessels.

Non-invasive imaging

Chest X-ray (CXR)

This simple investigation remains an important diagnostic tool in congenital heart disease.

- Advantages:
  - Cheap, widely available.
  - Enables serial comparison.
- Disadvantages:
  - Radiation dose.
  - Structures are projected in 2D and can be superimposed.

Points to look for:

- Extra cardiac—bones: cervical ribs, previous thoracotomy, kyphoscoliosis.
- Prosthetic material—clips coils, prosthetic valves, devices, sternal wires (not always used post-sternotomy in children).
- Situs—gastric bubble (normally L-sided), cardiac apex (normally to the L), bronchial pattern (long L and short R main bronchus) (囲 see pp.7–9.)
- Cardiothoracic ratio (CTR).
- Cardiac silhouette, typical patterns e.g.:
  - Pulmonary atresia—coeur en sabot (clog-shaped heart) (囲 see Fig. 2.3).
  - Ebstein—large globular heart (measure serial CTR) (囲 see Fig. 2.4).
  - Transposition of the great arteries (TGA)—'egg lying on its side' and narrow mediastinum (due to great vessels lying in an anteroposteriorly to each other) (Fig. 2.6).
- Calcification of e.g. conduits.
- Aortic arch:
  - R-sided arch may be identified.
  - Abnormal aortic knuckle or collaterals in coarctation.
- Pulmonary arteries (PA):
  - Any dilatation of PAs.
  - Absent PAs.
- Lung vascular markings:
  - Pulmonary blood flow—plethoric or oligaemic lung fields.
  - Abnormal vascular pattern suggesting abnormal PA or pulmonary vein (PV) anatomy.
  - Dilated abnormal vessels may represent major aortopulmonary collateral arteries (MAPCAs) (囲 see Pulmonary atresia with VSD, p.168).
  - Enlarged peripheral vessels may be pulmonary arteriovenous malformations.
- Lung parenchyma—Evidence of additional pulmonary disease.

Examples of the structures seen on P–A and lateral CXRs are illustrated in Figs. 2.1–2.7.

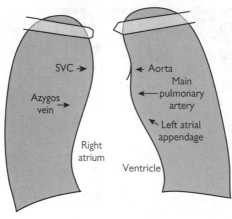

Fig. 2.1 P–A CXR—anatomical landmarks.

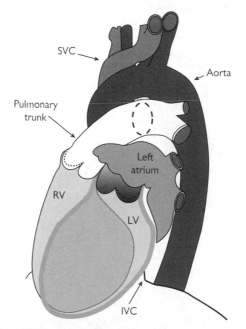

Fig. 2.2 Lateral CXR—anatomical landmarks.

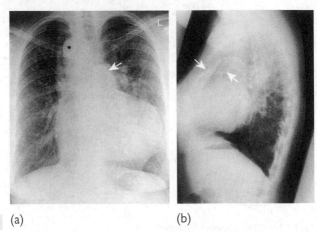

(a)   (b)

Fig. 2.3 Chest radiographs, (a) posteroanterior and (b) lateral, of a 30-year-old woman with tetralogy of Fallot and pulmonary atresia who underwent repair with a valved homograft conduit from right ventricle to pulmonary artery and ventricular septal defect closure 10 years previously. There is a right aortic arch (*) and a 'coeur en sabot' cardiac silhouette. The calcification in the homograft (arrows) is more clearly seen on the lateral radiograph. The abnormal pulmonary vasculature reflects persisting aortopulmonary collaterals. Reproduced from Warrell, D et al., (2005). *Oxford Textbook of Medicine* 4th edn, with permission from Oxford University Press.

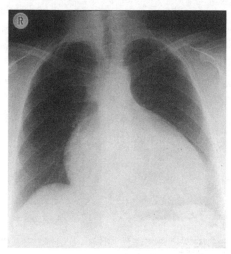

Fig. 2.4 Ebstein's anomaly with globular cardiomegaly due to dilated RA.

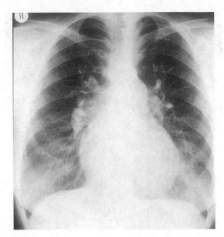

Fig. 2.5 Eisenmenger ASD—enlarged central PAs and pruning of distal vessels to give oligaemic lung fields.

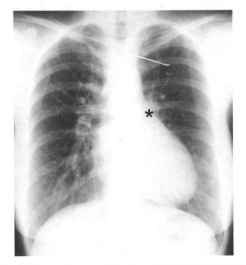

Fig. 2.6 Transposition of the great arteries. The cardiac mass has an 'egg on its side' appearance. There is a narrow mediastinum: the aorta lies directly anterior to the PA. The L heart border is straightened as the ascending aorta arises from the R ventricular outflow tract (*).

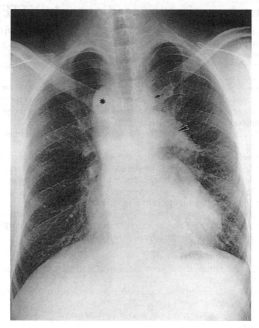

Fig. 2.7 Tetralogy of Fallot palliated with a classical left Blalock–Taussig shunt (small arrow). There is 2° dilatation of the LPA (large arrow) and a R aortic arch (*). Reproduced from Warrell D, Cox TM, Firth JM, *et al.* (eds) (2003). *Oxford Textbook of Medicine* 4th edn, p.1091, with permission from Oxford University Press.

Transthoracic echocardiography (TTE)

- Portable and widely available imaging tool which is safe, particularly for serial imaging.
- However:
  - Experience is essential when imaging patients with congenital heart disease and studies are operator dependent.
  - Some patients, especially after surgery may have difficult acoustic windows and there may be limited views of anterior structures.
- A sequential segmental approach should be used in all patients, especially if complex disease (📕 see Sequential segmental analysis, p.6).
  If difficulties in obtaining parasternal views, use an apical 4-chamber view.
- Patients may have >1 lesion.
- Basic echocardiography principles should be applied: assessment of ventricular function using dimensions and quantitative assessment including Simpson's rule, mitral annular planar systolic excursion (MAPSE), tricuspid annular planar systolic excursion (TAPSE), tissue Doppler velocities and myocardial performance index.
- New techniques that should improve the assessment of the patient with congenital heart disease include speckle tracking, strain imaging, 3D echo and assessment of dyssynchrony.

Particular strengths of TTE

- Anatomical assessment of ventricular, atrial, and valvular structure, function (Fig 2.9).
- Doppler measures of flow across valves, coarctation, shunt calculations/ gradients (Fig 2.8).
- Tissue Doppler assessment of ventricular function.
- Stress echo particularly in arterial switch patients.
- Contrast echo for identification of shunts.
- Assessment of baffle leaks or obstruction.
- Identification of PVs.
- 3D assessment of valvular structure and function, particularly in Ebstein's anomaly.

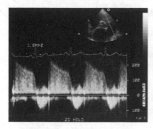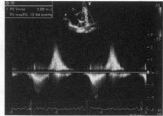

Fig. 2.8 Doppler assessment of mild (L) pulmonary regurgitation and severe (R) pulmonary regurgitation in patients with repaired tetralogy of Fallot.

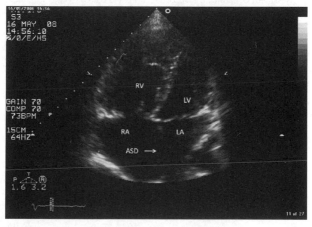

Fig. 2.9 Apical 4-chamber—secundum ASD with dilated RV.

Transoesophageal echo (TOE)

- Requires experienced hands for congenital heart disease patients—operator dependent.
- Excellent views of intracardiac structures e.g. complex outflow tracts, valve anatomy, posterior structures e.g. abnormal or post surgical PVs, atrial septum.
- Of particular use perioperatively.
- A sequential segmental approach should be followed in all patients (🕮 see Sequential segmental analysis, p.6).

Roles of TOE

- Ventricular function.
- PVs (Fig 2.11).
- Valvular structure and function, especially the adequacy of valve repair.
- Assessment of cardiovascular connections, intracardiac repairs, shunts (Fig 2.12).
- Guiding and periprocedural ASD/VSD/PFO/baffle leak closure.
- Intraoperative assessment of ventricular and valular function, haemodynamics, adequacy of valve repairs or replacements and surgical reconstructions.
- Assessment of intracardiac thrombus/mass and prior to cardioversion.
- Provides diagnostic information on patients with limited TTE views following previous surgery or chest deformities.
- Excellent visualization of complications of Fontan procedure (Fig. 2.10) e.g. obstruction or thrombosis.
- Visualization of atrial baffles to detect stenoses or leaks.
- Provides evaluation of AV valves and site of chordal insertion.
- Characterizes outflow tract obstructions, abnormalities of the aorta, such as CoA and PDA.

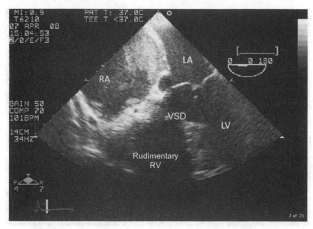

Fig. 2.10 Fontan (tricuspid atresia, TGA) with spontaneous echo contrast in the Fontan pathway (RA).

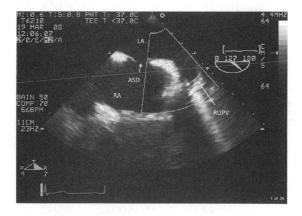

Fig. 2.11 Secundum ASD demonstrating R upper PV (RUPV).

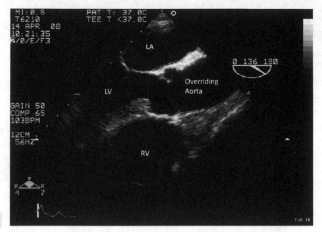

Fig. 2.12 Repaired tetralogy of Fallot demonstrating the aorta overriding the crest of the interventricular septum (*).

Cardiovascular magnetic resonance (CMR) imaging

- Gold standard method for the characterization of cardiac anatomy, function, and mass.
- Provides clear anatomical images throughout the chest.
- Accurate and reliable technique for serial monitoring of patients, particularly in response to therapeutic intervention.
- No radiation—particularly relevant to young patients with long life-expectancy who require multiple scans over many years.
- Increasing availability.

Disadvantages, cautions, and contraindications

- Expensive.
- Requires specialist training.
- Potentially lengthy scans and breath-holds.
- Echo provides better images of fine mobile structures e.g. valves and atrial septum.
- Some patients (2%) are claustrophobic.
- Susceptibility artefacts from stents, sternal wires, and rods from spinal deformities.
- Pacemakers, ICDs, aneurysm clips, or metallic implants are *contraindicated*.

Gadolinium contrast

- IV gadolinium contrast can be used to provide 3D contrast angiography, assess myocardial viability or the presence of scar tissue.
- Care should be used with contrast in certain patients with impaired renal function (NICE Guidelines 2007).[1]

Role of MRI in congenital heart disease

- L and R ventricular volumes, mass, and function e.g. repaired tetralogy of Fallot patients prior to pulmonary valve replacement (Fig 2.13).
- Assessment of valvar regurgitant volume and fraction.
- Coarctation and aortic disease:
  - Aorta and arch anatomy.
  - Native coarctation or recoarctation, peak velocity, and evidence of diastolic tail, collaterals (with 3D gadolinium contrast angiography).
  - Serial assessment of aneurysms (Fig. 2.17) and dilated aorta.
- Anomalous vascular branches and collaterals using 3D gadolinium contrast angiography e.g. anomalous pulmonary venous drainage.
- Assessment of shunts e.g. PDA, ASD, VSD by measuring the difference between pulmonary and aortic flows.
- Monitoring of operated patients: assessment of pulmonary artery stenoses e.g. conduit patency, venous pathway patency e.g. Mustard and Senning patients (Figs. 2.14, 2.15), tetralogy of Fallot (Fig. 2.16), Fontan connections (Fig. 2.18).

---

1 NICE (2007). Available at: http://www.nice.org.uk/nicemedia/pdf/CG64NICEguidance.pdf.

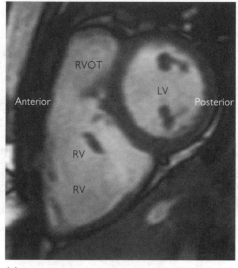

(a)

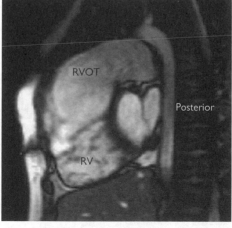

(b)

Fig. 2.13 Short-axis cardiac MR of a patient with tetralogy of Fallot showing (a) a dilated right ventricle and (b) a dilated RV patch outflow tract.

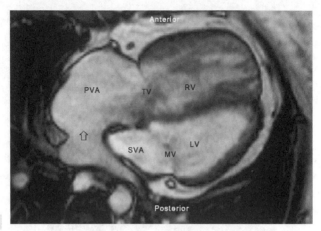

Fig. 2.14 TGA/Mustard with systemic RV and widely open pulmonary venous pathway. LV left ventricle; MV mitral valve; PVA pulmonary venous atrium; RV right ventricle; SVA systemic venous atrium; TV tricuspid valve.

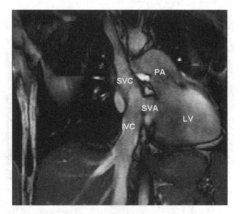

Fig. 2.15 TGA/Mustard with subpulmonary LV and widely patent systemic venous pathway. IVC inferior vena cava; LV left ventricle; PA pulmonary artery; SVA systemic venous atrium; SVC superior vena cava.

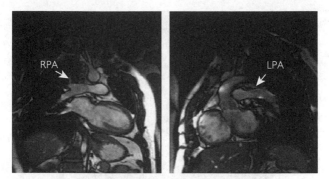

Fig. 2.16 Widely patent R and L pulmonary arteries in a repaired tetralogy of Fallot patient.

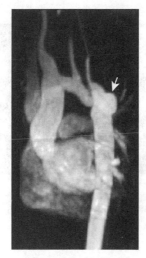

Fig. 2.17 Aneursym formation (white arrow) at a coarctation surgical repair site.

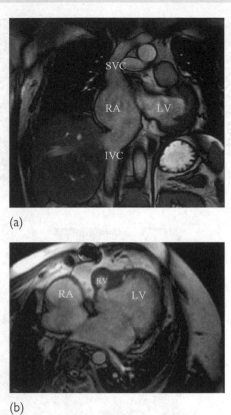

(a)

(b)

Fig. 2.18 (a) Fontan pathway with SVC and IVC entering RA and (b) dominant LV and rudimentary RV.

Computed tomography (CT)

- Provides very high resolution imaging particularly of coronary arteries, collateral vessels, aorta, lung, pericardial calcification.
- Advanced imaging modality of choice in patients with
  - Contraindications to MRI e.g. pacemakers, ICDs.
  - Prosthetic materials that cause MRI image degradation e.g. coarctation stent, spinal rods.

Disadvantages

- The ionizing radiation dose limits repeated usage.
- Caution if using contrast in patients with impaired renal function.

Particular uses

- Anomalous coronary arteries
- Coarctation stent follow-up (see Plate II).
- Assessment of cardiovascular connections and great vessel relations (🕮 see Fig 2.19).
- Course of collateral vessels.
- Evidence of coronary and pericardial calcification.
- Patients with contraindications to MRI.

Recommended reading

Ayres NA, Miller-Hance W, Fyfe DA, et al. (2005). Indications and guidelines for performance of transesophageal echocardiography in the patient with pediatric acquired or congenital heart disease: report from the task force of the Pediatric Council of the American Society of Echocardiography. *J Am Soc Echocardiogr* **18**(1), 91–8.

Crean A (2007). Cardiovascular MR and CT in congenital heart disease. *Heart* **93**, 1637–47.

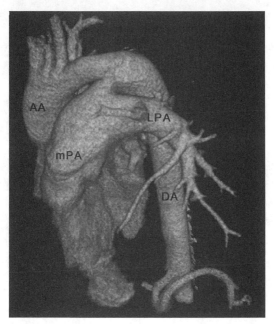

Fig. 2.19 (📖 See Plate 12) Eisenmenger PDA. 3D reconstruction from multi-slice CT scan demonstrating a PDA (arrow) in a 36-year-old woman with Eisenmenger syndrome. AA ascending aorta; DA descending aorta; LPA and mPA left and main pulmonary artery.

Physiological testing

Physiological testing

Introduction
Exercise testing provides objective evidence of performance in cardiac disease. There are many testing protocols available but they usually involve incremental increase in exercise either on a treadmill or an exercise bike. Metabolic or cardiopulmonary exercise testing (CPEX) measures ventilation and the inspired and expired oxygen (O_2) and carbon dioxide (CO_2) levels during graded exercise to objectively assess performance. It is possible to derive the maximum oxygen uptake (VO_2 max), anaerobic threshold (AT) and VE/VCO_2 slope all of which give prognostic information. When combined with pulmonary function testing, CPEX is a very useful tool in assessing the contribution of cardiac condition to breathlessness.

Indications for exercise testing
- Determine cause of clinical deterioration.
- Determine cause of breathlessness.
- Detect exercise-induced arrhythmia.
- Assess need for, and effect of, interventions.
- Work-up for heart (and lung) transplantation.
- Pre-pregnancy assessment.
- Assess suitability for competitive and leisure sports.

Testing procedures
Even for seemingly low-risk individuals, full resuscitation facilities must be available before exercise testing is performed.

Types of exercise tests

6-minute walk

- Simple, self paced test, may stop to rest.
- Most useful for very limited patients, where it acts as a maximal test:
  - <450m 6-minute walk distance correlates well with symptoms and peak VO_2.
- Limited by inter-test variability—very important to standardize methods used.

Bruce exercise test (or similar)

- Available in most hospitals.
- Incremental exercise, increase in speed and slope.
- Continuous ECG monitoring for ST segment changes.
- Very useful if ischaemic heart disease suspected.
- Unable to determine if anaerobic threshold reached.
- Prognostic information for risk of future coronary events only (low risk in congenital heart disease).

Metabolic (cardiopulmonary) exercise testing (CPEX)

- Objective assessment of performance based on incremental exercise and analysis of inspired and expired O_2 and CO_2.
- Can perform full lung function tests at same time.
- Gives prognostic information, in terms of mortality risk in chronic heart failure.
- Can ensure maximal effort is performed by analysis of anaerobic threshold.
- Not universally available.
- Requires specialist knowledge for interpretation of results.

Bruce exercise testing

Many centres do not have facilities for metabolic exercise testing and standard Bruce exercise testing can be used to estimate the maximal O_2 consumption:

- Standard Bruce protocol with incremental increases and inclines.
- Exercise duration is measured in time expressed as decimal.
- Formulae as follows based on active and sedentary (i.e. non athletic), T = exercise duration in minutes (decimal):
  - ♂ VO_2 max $= 14.8 - (1.379 \times T) + (0.451 \times T^2) - (0.012 \times T^3)$ mL/kg/min.
  - ♀ VO_2 max $= 4.38 \times T - 3.9$ mL/kg/min.
- Doesn't provide evidence of maximal exercise or anaerobic threshold.

Metabolic exercise testing

Protocol
The exercise protocol should be:
- Maximal incremental (stair-step or ramp) test.
- Ideally 8–12min duration.

Treadmill or bicycle
- Advantage of treadmill is higher achievable maximal results (10–15%).
- Advantages with bicycle testing are:
  - More suitable in some patients with disability.
  - Less noise when monitoring exercise blood pressure (BP).

Measurements

Lung function
Restrictive lung defects due to previous thoracotomies or spinal abnormalities are common in congenital heart disease, therefore measure:
- Forced vital capacity—FVC.
- Forced expiratory volume in 1sec—FEV1.

Also consider:
- Body plethysmography.
- Total lung capacity—TLC.
- Vital capacity—VC.
- Diffusion capacity.

Exercise testing
The patient breathes through a mouthpiece or face mask to measure expired gases and respiratory effort continuously during exercise. The following are measured:
- Minute ventilation.
- Continuous gas exchange.
  - VO_2.
  - VCO_2.
- Continuous 12-lead ECG monitoring.
- BP.
- O_2 saturation.

Reports
The cardiopulmonary exercise report in adult congenital heart disease should contain the following information:
- Diagnosis/indication for testing.
- Exercise protocol used duration of exercise.
- Comments regarding lung function (normal/limited).
- ECG.
  - Maximum HR, HR at 1 and 2min post exercise.
  - Rhythm.
- BP.
  - At peak exercise or immediately post exercise.
- O_2 saturation (start and at peak/immediately after exercise).
- Exercise flow and metabolic gas exchange.
  - Maximum minute ventilation (V_E max).

- Maximum oxygen uptake (VO_2 max).
- Respiratory exchange ratio (RER) values >1 indicate anaerobic threshold (i.e. maximal exercise) has been reached.
- Comparison with expected values and with previous tests.
- Conclusion and consequences of the test.

Data derived from the test is displayed in a Wassermann nine-panel display. 📖 see Further reading.

Prognostic significance of results

Prognostic significance of results from metabolic exercise testing has been assessed in heart failure, but has not been verified in congenital heart disease. Nevertheless it does provide objective information on the cardiac and respiratory status of these patients.

In chronic heart failure prognosis (death within 18 months) is predicted by the following:
- VO_2 max <12mL/kg/min.
- AT <8mL/kg/min.
- VE/VCO_2 slope >34.

Where:
- AT = anaerobic threshold, the point at which aerobic respiration is supplemented by anaerobic respiration, with ↑ lactate production, and buffering with bicarbonate, detected by an increase in CO_2 output, measured in L/min or normalized to bodyweight (mL/kg/min).
- VCO_2 = CO_2 output, the amount of CO_2 exhaled from the body into the atmosphere per unit time, measured in L/min or normalized to bodyweight (mL/kg/min).
- VE = minute ventilation, the amount of gas exhaled divided by time in minutes for gas to be collected (L/min).
- VE/VCO_2 = ventilatory equivalent for CO_2.
- VO_2 = amount of O_2 extracted from the inspired gas in a given period of time measured in L/min or normalized to bodyweight (mL/kg/min).
- VO_2 max = the highest O_2 uptake obtainable for a given exercise despite further increases in work and effort.

Further reading

Wasserman K, Hansen JE, Sue DY, et al. (2004). *Principles or exercise testing and interpretation*. 4th edn. Lippincott Williams & Wilkins.

Cardiac catheterization

Introduction

The purpose of cardiac catheterization in this patient group is to gain information about complex anatomy and haemodynamics, especially with respect to PA pressure and vascular resistance. In order to gain complete angiographic and haemodynamic information, studies are best performed in specialist units. In recent years, catheterization has been increasingly combined with percutaneous interventional procedures, reducing the need for further cardiac surgery in some individuals. 📖 See Table 4.1 for a list of commonly used terms and abbreviations.

Table 4.1 Glossary of commonly used abbreviations

A–P	Antero-posterior
CI	Cardiac index
CO	Cardiac output
FA	Femoral artery
IVC	Inferior vena cava
LAO	Left anterior oblique
LAVV	Left atrioventricular valve
LV	Left ventricle
LVOT	Left ventricular outflow tract
mLA	Mean left atrial pressure
mRA	Mean right atrial pressure
mPAP	Mean pulmonary artery pressure
mPCWP	Mean pulmonary capillary wedge pressure
mSAP	Mean systolic arterial pressure
PA	Pulmonary artery
PR	Pulmonary regurgitation
PV	Pulmonary vein
PVR	Pulmonary vascular resistance
PVRI	Indexed pulmonary vascular resistance
QP	Pulmonary blood flow
QS	Systemic blood flow
RAO	Right anterior oblique
RAVV	Right atrioventricular valve
RV	Right ventricle
RVOT	Right ventricular outflow tract
RV–PA	Right ventricle to pulmonary artery
SVC	Superior vena cava
SVR	Systemic vascular resistance
SVRI	Indexed systemic vascular resistance
TOE	Transoesophageal echocardiogram
VSD	Ventricular septal defect

Indications for catheterization

Secundum atrial septal defect
- Device closure during same procedure.
- Shunt calculation ± coronary angiography if unsuitable for device closure.

Coarctation (re-coarctation or native)
- Measure gradient—care in passing through coarctation, consider radial approach to gain ascending aortic pressure.
- Demonstrate anatomy— RAO and lateral projections (arms above head) to demonstrate coarctation.
- Consider crossing aortic valve for pullback gradient (80% bicuspid aortic valve).
- Dilation and stent deployment.

Post tetralogy of Fallot repair
- RV function.
- Degree of PR.
- Branch PA stenosis (and dilation and stenting).
- LV function and residual VSD.
- Coronary disease in older patient.

RV–PA conduit
- Assess conduit function.

Atrioventricular septal defect
- Look for L atrioventricular valve incompetence regurgitation.
- Elongated LVOT so care in measuring pullback gradient (sub-valvar stenosis).
- Calculate shunt in unoperated cases.

Fontan
- Angiography in Fontan pathway to demonstrate pathway stenosis with follow through to look for pulmonary venous return and collaterals.
- Small pressure gradients are significant, ensure zeros are correct.
- Measure ventricular end-diastolic pressure.
- Estimate pulmonary vascular resistance.

Post Mustard or Senning operation for TGA
- Atrial pathway obstruction (and dilation and stenting).
- Atrial baffle leaks (and device occlusion).
- Systemic ventricular function and atrioventricular valve regurgitation.
- Pulmonary vascular resistance.

Precatheterization care

- If cyanosed or complex congenital heart disease, especially Fontan and pulmonary hypertension (PHT): pre-hydrate whilst NBM with 1 L normal saline over 12 hours to prevent contrast induced nephropathy and reduce risk of circulatory collapse.
- Stop warfarin 2 days prior to procedure and heparinize if necessary.
- If under general anaesthesia ensure experienced anesthetist.
- Consent for ~1% risk of significant complications including death.
- In ♀ of child bearing age ensure −ve pregnancy test.
- Height and weight are recorded.
- Shave both groins (may have had previous cutdowns).

Choice of catheters

Left heart catheterization

- Standard Judkins catheters are generally all that is necessary for L-heart catheterization. Anomalous origins of the coronary arteries are more common in congenital heart disease and therefore, Williams R coronary catheter or modified Amplatz right coronary (MARC) catheters may be necessary to locate the R coronary ostium.
- Ventricular angiography is best performed using a pigtail catheter, however if following ventriculography an accurate pullback gradient is necessary through the ventricular outflow tract then exchange for an end-hole catheter such as a Judkins right 4 catheter or Multipurpose A1 (MPA1).

Right heart catheterization

- In congenital heart disease this requires a high level of expertise. The positioning of catheters in the R heart can be difficult owing to the altered anatomy in repaired hearts, chamber dilatation, or the abnormal position of the outflow tract (e.g. congenitally corrected transposition of the great arteries (ccTGA) or post Rastelli operation).
- For haemodynamic studies the experienced operator will usually use a 6F MPA1 or MPB3 catheter as these catheters are very manoeuvrable; alternatively a Judkins JR4 catheter may suffice. Care must be taken to avoid inducing arrhythmias, and pressure injections must not be given through single end-hole catheters.
- For angiography, a catheter with side holes is required and that includes the MPB3 (Gensini) and the Pigtail, NIA, or Berman flotation catheters. The advantage of the pigtail catheter is that catheter recoil is less likely during pump angiography. The disadvantage of the NIA and Berman catheters is that neither have an end hole and therefore a guide wire cannot be used to position or exchange the catheter, and a wedge trace cannot be obtained. The benefit of the Berman catheter is that it is a balloon flotation catheter and it may be possible to float the catheter around a difficult subpulmonary ventricle without inducing arrhythmias.
- Remember that if a patient is cyanotic then the balloon should not be filled with air as balloon rupture will lead to an air embolus. The balloon can be filled instead with CO_2 which will dissolve rapidly in the event of balloon rupture.

- In order to minimize the risk of catheter recoil during angiography in the PAs and subpulmonary ventricle, consider using a lower flow rate at lower pressure and with a transition time of 1sec (e.g. 30mL of contrast at 10mL per sec, at 600psi with 1sec transition.
- Routine assessments of cardiac catheterization

Oxygen saturations
- Always—IVC, SVC, PA, FA.
- If necessary—RA/RV/LV/PV.

Pressure measurements (ensure zero is correct)
- RA (a wave, v wave, and mean), RV (systolic and EDP) PA (systolic, diastolic, and mean), PCWP (a wave, v wave, and mean).
- FA (systolic, diastolic, mean), aortic (systolic, diastolic, mean), and LV (systolic, diastolic, mean).

Angiography
Ventricular angiography
- To assess function, outflow tracts, and atrioventricular valve regurgitation.
- RV (AP and lateral planes).
- LV (RAO and LAO/cranial planes). Interventricular septum best profiled in LV LAO/cranial view.

Aortography
- RAO 45° and LAO 45° projections.
- Purpose—to assess root dimensions degree of aortic incompetence, coarctation site, aortopulmonary shunts, collateral vessels, anomalous coronary arteries.

Pulmonary arteriography
- RAO and LAO cranial planes.
- RAO projection profiles the proximal RPA.
- LAO cranial projection profiles the proximal LPA.
- Use AP cranial projection for bifurcation stenoses.

Coronary angiography
If coronary disease suspected/precardiac surgery if risk factors for coronary disease. Coronary anomalies are common; initial aortogram may indicate anomalous coronary origin.

Calculations

Shunt calculation by oximetry

- Mixed venous saturation = $(3 \times SVC + IVC) / 4$.
- QP/QS = (Ao sat – mixed venous sat)/(PV sat – PA sat).

Cardiac output (CO)

- O_2 consumption (VO_2) estimated at 3mL/kg or measured.
- Arterio-venous oxygen difference (AVO_2) = arterial –mixed venous O_2 content.
- O_2 content = sats $\times$ 1.36 $\times$ Hb.
- CO = O_2 consumption / ($AVO_2 \times 10$) (NR 4–8L/min).
- CO = (wt $\times$ 3) / ((arterial sats – mixed venous sats) $\times$ 1.36 $\times$ Hb $\times$ 10).
- CI = CO/BSA (NR 2.5–4.2L/min/m^2)

Systemic vascular resistance

- SVR = (mSAP – mRA) / CO (NR 10–14) Wood units.
- SVRI = (mSAP– mRA) / CI (NR 25-30).
- Multiply $\times$ 80 for SVR in dynes.sec/cm^5 (NR 700–1600) and SVRI in dyne.sec/cm^5/m^2 (NR 1970–2390).

Pulmonary vascular resistance

- Transpulmonary gradient (TPG) = mPAP – mLAP (mPCWP).
- PVR (in Wood units) = TPG/CO (NR 1–4).
- PVRI = TPG/CI (NR 3–4).
- Multiply $\times$ 80 for PVR in dynes.sec/cm^5 (NR <250) and PVRI in dyne.sec/cm^5/m^2 (NR 255–285).

Influence of pulmonary blood flow on management and outcome

Introduction

Delivery of systemic venous blood to the alveolar capillary membrane to allow release of waste CO_2 and uptake of O_2 depends on the integrity of the pulmonary circulation. Too little blood flow to the lungs and the patient is hypoxic; too much and the lungs become oedematous.

Pulmonary vascular development in early life

Fetal circulation

In the fetal circulation the pulmonary arterial tree is muscular and non-compliant. This leads to very high pulmonary vascular resistances *in utero*, necessary to divert the oxygenated blood returning from the umbilical vein to bypass the lungs and run into the systemic circulation *via* the ductus arteriosus.

At birth, the newborn child inflates the lungs for the 1st time and blood is drawn into the pulmonary circulation, filling it for the 1st time. The ↑ pulmonary venous return raises the L atrial pressure and the foramen ovale closes. The flow through the ductus arteriosus reverses stimulating the contraction and closure of this communication in the first few days of life, thus establishing the pulmonary and systemic circulations.

Normal pulmonary vascular development

- The muscular pulmonary arterial tree changes in the 1st few months of life:
  - The smooth muscle layer of the pulmonary arterial tree recedes from the capillary level back to the larger pulmonary arteries →
  - The pulmonary arterioles, the resistance vessels of the lungs, become non-muscular, highly compliant elastic vessels (properties that are retained throughout life) →
  - Permits large changes in cardiac output (e.g. during exercise), without any appreciable change in PAP.
- If a child's lungs are exposed to high pressure and flow in the neonatal period (e.g. large VSD), then these changes in pulmonary vasculature do not occur. Instead, progressive pulmonary vascular remodelling takes place, → PHT if the defect is not repaired (Fig. 5.1)

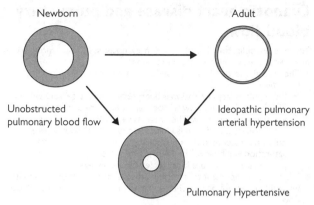

Fig. 5.1 Pulmonary vascular remodelling

Cyanotic heart disease and pulmonary blood flow

There is an obligatory R-to-L shunt in cyanosis: systemic venous blood mixes with the systemic arterial circulation.
- The critical question in a cyanosed patient is *what is the pulmonary blood flow?*
  - If the pulmonary circulation is unprotected (e.g. large VSD with no PS) then pulmonary flow will be high, at high pressure. Pulmonary vascular remodelling will be progressive and PHT will occur.
  - If pulmonary blood flow is limited (e.g. large VSD with severe pulmonary stenosis) then pulmonary flow and systemic arterial saturation will be low. The PA pressure will be low i.e. the pulmonary vasculature is protected by the presence of PS.
- It is critically important to determine the pulmonary blood flow as it will guide intervention to either decrease or increase pulmonary blood flow.

Determining pulmonary blood flow
- TTE may be sufficient to assess pulmonary flow in the neonate.
- Cardiac catheterization may be necessary.
- In pulmonary atresia (no pulmonary outflow from heart) the pulmonary blood flow is dependent on either:
  - Collateral vessels, called major aortopulmonary collateral arteries (MAPCAs) (📖 see p.168).

or

  - Persistence of the ductus arteriosus. If the duct closes a precipitous and perilous fall in pulmonary blood flow will occur with associated fall in systemic saturations. The duct is therefore kept open until surgical intervention using an infusion of prostaglandin E1 (Prostin®).

Restricting pulmonary blood flow
- In order to limit unobstructed pulmonary blood flow, the PA is surgically banded.
- Protects distal pulmonary circulation from high pressure flow whilst allowing adequate oxygenation.
- The band is usually removed at later definitive surgery.
- Adults who had a PA band removed in childhood may have mild pulmonary arterial stenosis at the site of the band.

Increasing pulmonary blood flow

- If pulmonary blood flow is inadequate in early life it may be enhanced by a surgical shunt (📖 see Fig. 5.2) or pulmonary valvotomy (transcatheter or surgical). Shunt operations include:
  - Classical Blalock–Taussig (BT) shunt—subclavian to PA anastomosis (historical, no longer used).
  - Modified BT shunt—a Gore-tex® tube placed between subclavian and PAs.
  - Central shunt—Gore-tex® tube between innominate and PAs.
  - Waterston shunt—direct communication between AA and RPA (historical, no longer used).
  - Potts anastomosis—direct communication between DA and LPA (historical, no longer used).
- After 4–6 months of life, PVR has usually fallen sufficiently to allow augmentation of pulmonary blood supply by a systemic venous-to-pulmonary artery shunt:
  - The Glenn (cavo-pulmomary) shunt is a connection between the SVC and PA (📖 see Fig. 5.3)
    —classical Glenn: side-to-end anastomosis between SVC and RPA with RPA disconnected from MPA.
    —bidirectional Glenn: end-to-side anastomosis between SVC and RPA. RPA remains in continuity with main and LPA.
  - In childhood, the SVC return accounts for 70% of venous return, so a Glenn shunt provides adequate oxygenation. An adult with a Glenn as the sole source of pulmonary blood supply will be deeply cyanosed because SVC return is only ~25% of venous return.
  - Pulmonary arteriovenous-malformations often develop late after a Glenn shunt, causing ↑ R-to-L shunting through lungs and ↑ cyanosis, plus risk of pulmonary haemorrhage.
- In an obligatory R-to-L shunt, normal pulmonary blood flow is indicated by systemic arterial shunts of ~85%. Higher values suggest ↑ pulmonary blood flow and lower values insufficient pulmonary blood flow.

Summary

If pulmonary blood flow is unobstructed at high pressure due to a cardiac defect, then blood flow to lungs needs limiting in neonatal life to prevent pulmonary vascular remodelling. If pulmonary blood flow is insufficient then a systemic arterial or venous to PA shunt is required to maintain systemic arterial saturations and normal growth of the child.

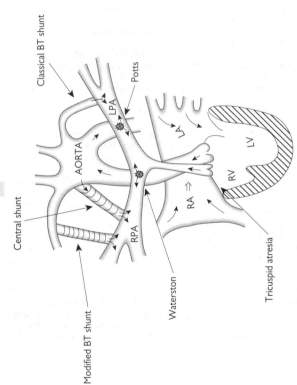

Fig. 5.2 (📖 See also Plate 1) Types of systemic–pulmonary arterial shunts (tricuspid atresia).

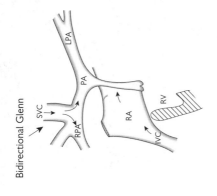

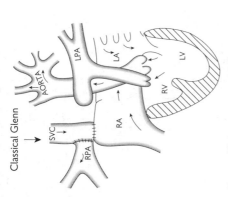

Fig. 5.3 (□ See also Plate 2) Systemic venous-to-pulmonary arterial shunts—the Glenn anastomosis.

Cyanosis

Introduction

Cyanosis is only present where there is a R-to-L shunt. The shunt may be anywhere e.g. intracardiac, between great vessels, intrapulmonary. Cyanosis is usually clinically detectable at SaO_2 <85%. Cyanosis may be associated with low, normal, or high pulmonary blood flow or pulmonary vascular resistance (see p.52).

All cyanotic patients should be seen at a specialist centre.

Non-cardiac manifestations of cyanosis

- Blood and vessels (see following sections for more detail):
  - Erythrocytosis 2° to hypoxia.
  - Thrombocytopenia.
  - Coagulopathy; haemorrhage or thrombosis.
  - Fe deficiency 2° to over-venesection or menorrhagia.
  - Atherosclerotic coronary (and other systemic arterial) disease is exceedingly rare.
- Neurological:
  - Cerebrovascular accident (CVA) 2° to paradoxical embolism.
  - Cerebral abscess.
- Renal impairment:
  - Due to glomerular proteinuria, mesangial matrix thickening, capillary and hilar arteriole dilatation.
  - → risk of iatrogenic renal failure if dehydration, aminoglycosides, NSAIA, intravascular contrast agents.
- Gout.
- Pigment gallstones.
- Acne.
- Digital clubbing.
- Hypertrophic osteoarthropathy.

Secondary erythrocytosis (polycythaemia)

This is a physiological adaptation to hypoxia, maximizing O_2-carrying capacity. It may cause symptomatic hyperviscosity, but is not a contributory factor to the ↑ risk of stroke seen in patients with cyanotic heart disease.

Venesection to reduce haematocrit

- Should not be done routinely, it does not reduce the risk of stroke.
- May cause cardiovascular collapse if simultaneous volume replacement is not given.
- May cause Fe deficiency, which increases the risk of stroke.
- Should only be performed for temporary relief of symptoms of hyperviscosity.

📖 See Table 6.1.

Table 6.1 Guidelines for venesection in cyanotic congenital heart disease

Symptoms of hyperviscosity	Haematocrit and serum Fe	Action
No	Any	Venesection not indicated
Yes	Hct >60%	Isovolumic venesection (400–500mL)
	Fe replete	
	No dehydration	
Yes	Hct <65%	Treat underlying cause of Fe deficiency No venesection
	Fe deficient	Consider low dose Fe therapy, closely monitoring Hct
Yes	>65%	Seek underlying cause of Fe deficiency
	Fe deficient	Avoid venesection if possible
		Consider cautious low dose
		Fe ± hydroxyurea

Coagulation

- Risk of major haemorrhage:
  - Surgery.
  - Haemoptysis, especially if PHT or collaterals.
- PA thrombosis *in situ* if PHT:
  - Associated with PA atherosclerotic changes.
  - Risk increases with age.
  - May embolize to peripheral PAs → ↑ hypoxia and cyanosis.
  - Anticoagulation often ineffective in resolving PA thrombus.
- Warfarin anticoagulation:
  - Difficult—individualize decision; risk of bleeding *vs.* risk of thromboembolism.
  - Control difficult—spuriously high INR results if Hct >55 unless amount of citrate anticoagulant in sample bottle reduced.

$$\text{Vol. citrate per mL blood} = \frac{100 - \text{Hct}}{595 - \text{Hct}}$$

Checklist for inpatients and emergencies with cyanotic heart disease

Avoid iatrogenic renal dysfunction
- No NSAIAs.
- Aminoglycosides only with great care.
- IV fluids when NBM or intravascular contrast agents.

Reduce risk of paradoxical embolism
- Use air filters on IV lines.
- Use infusion pumps with bubble detector.

Maintain adequate Hb post op for optimum O_2-carrying capacity

Avoid vasodilators—they increase cyanosis.

Tachyarrhythmias
- Atrial arrhythmias often atypical—patients should be provided with a copy of their ECG in sinus rhythm (SR) to carry with them, so easy comparison can be made.
- Atrial arrhythmias often poorly tolerated—prompt restoration of SR required.
- DC cardioversion often safer than acute drug therapy.

Haemoptysis
- May be life threatening—admit.
- IV fluids, X match blood, FFP, platelets.
- CT to identify site of bleeding.
- If Eisenmenger, remember brachial artery BP is same as PA pressure. Treat systemic hypertension with β blocker (do not use vasodilator). Sedation may be needed.
- Bleeding collaterals may be possible to embolize—transfer to specialist centre.
- Major bleeding—consider selective intubation of non-bleeding lung.
- Catastrophic bleeding likely to be fatal—high dose opiates appropriate.

Cerebral abscess
- Suspect if unexplained fever, leucoctyosis, headache, or new neurological signs.
- Urgent contrast enhanced CT and blood cultures.
- NB cerebral abscess may be presenting complaint in cyanotic disease: e.g. pulmonary AVM, anomalous systemic venous drainage.
- Cyanosis should be sought in all cases of cerebral abscess. L-arm bubble contrast echo to confirm (R-arm injection will miss any anomalously draining persistent LSVC).

Part 2

Specific lesions

Valve and outflow tract lesions

Left ventricular outflow tract obstruction (LVOTO)

Introduction

LVOTO may occur at different levels:
- Subvalvular.
- Valvular—including bicuspid aortic valve.
- Supravalvular.
- Coarctation—📖 see p.118.

Effects of LVOTO, irrespective of site of lesion, are:
- ↑ afterload on LV.
- LV hypertrophy.
- Eventual LV dilatation and failure.

Subvalvar aortic stenosis (AS)

Definition and incidence
- Obstruction due to either:
  - Discrete fibromuscular or membranous subvalvar ridge (90%), *or*
  - Fibromuscular tunnel.
- 6.5% of adults with congenital heart disease.
- ♂ predominance (2:1).
- Usually sporadic but familial cases reported.

Associations
- Mitral valve (MV) anomalies.
- AVSD, VSD.
- Shone syndrome.

Natural history and presentation
- Stenosis is progressive but rate of progression is variable.
- May cause functional disruption of aortic valve → aortic regurgitation (AR), which may progress, even after resection of membrane.
- Presentation—as other causes of LVOTO.

Investigation and management
- Echo delineates anatomy and severity of obstruction as well as AR and associated lesions
- Surgical repair indicated if symptomatic, or mean gradient >50mmHg, LV dysfunction, progressive AR.
- Long-term follow up needed because:
  - Up to 37% recurrence risk, especially in tunnel-like lesions or if resting preoperative gradient >40mmHg.
  - Risk of progressive AR, despite surgical repair.

Bicuspid aortic valve

Definition and incidence
- Aortic valve comprises 2 cusps, often of unequal size.
- Commonest congenital cardiac anomaly—1–2% of population.
- ♂ predominance (4:1).
- May be inherited or sporadic.

Associations
- Co-existing aortopathy of ascending aorta →
  - Aortic root dilatation.
  - Risk of dissection.
- 20% have other anomalies e.g. coarctation, patent arterial duct.

Natural history and presentation
- Range of severity:
  - Severe *in utero* AS → failure of L heart to develop (hypoplastic L heart).
  - Severe AS requiring surgical repair as neonate.
  - Chance finding in late adulthood.
- Clinically important sequelae in adult—progressive AS, AR, and aortic root dilatation.
- Probability for AVR increases from 1% at 1–9 years to 30% at 60–69 years.

Investigation and management
Key points
- Symptoms occur late in young people, so regular follow up important.
- CXR—dilatation of ascending aorta (AA).
- ECG—LVH and left axis deviation if severe AS.
- Echo to monitor AV function, LV dimensions and function, associated anomalies.
- Exercise testing (medically supervised) in moderate-to-severe asymptomatic AS—intervene if ST segment changes, failure of BP to rise.
- Serial MRI if aortic root dilation.

Intervention
- Timing:
  - *AS:*
    —if symptoms and moderate–severe AS.
    —asymptomatic if: severe AS (mean gradient >50mmHg), impaired LV or abnormal exercise.
  - *AR:*
    —if symptoms and moderate-to-severe AR.
    —asymptomatic if progressive LV dilation or LV impairment.
- Balloon valvuloplasty only rarely indicated in adults—if minimal calcification and favourable valve morphology.
- Aortic valve replacement. Choice of valve depends on lifestyle, plans for childbearing, coexisting lesions.

Supravalvar AS

- Rarest form of LVOTO.
- Focal or diffuse narrowing; starts at sinotubular junction and may involve entire AA.
- Due to mutation of elastin gene on chromosome 7q11.23

Associations

- Most commonly seen in Williams syndrome.
- Familial forms and rare sporadic cases also reported.
- Aortic valve abnormalities in up to 50%, most commonly bicuspid valve.

Natural history and presentation

- Coronary involvement → worse prognosis than other forms of LVOTO:
  - Fibromuscular thickening may encroach into coronary ostia.
  - Coronaries lie proximal to obstruction so coronary circulation exposed to high LV pressures.
- Presentation—as other forms of LVOTO.
- May have associated signs of Williams syndrome (elfin-like face, short stature, low IQ). Stenosing arteriopathy in Williams syndrome may involve any artery including abdominal aorta and PAs.

Investigation and management

Key points

- Echo—anatomy and severity of supravalvar stenosis.
- MRI/CT—assess involvement of whole aorta and pulmonary tree.
- Cardiac catheter—assess severity of stenoses and coronary involvement.
- Surgical repair if symptoms, coronary involvement, or mean pressure gradient >50mmHg.

Left ventricular inflow lesions

Congenital mitral valve abnormalities

- Rare, usually stenotic.
- Usually associated with other cardiac defects:
  - L-sided obstructive defects (most commonly).
  - ASD, VSD, tetralogy of Fallot.

Types

Supra-mitral ring
- Membrane in LA immediately above MV, inferior to appendage (*cf.* cor triatriatum where membrane is superior to appendage).
- Membrane obstructs MV and may restrict leaflet motion.

Parachute mitral valve
- Papillary muscles either fused or 1 is absent/hypoplastic.
- Valve and subvalvar apparatus often dysplastic.
- Obstruction occurs at the level of the papillary muscles.

Mitral arcade
Absent or shortened chordae causing restricted leaflet mobility.

Double orifice mitral valve
- 2 orifices arise from excessive leaflet tissue.
- May cause restricted excursion of mitral leaflets.

Presentation
- Majority diagnosed and repaired in childhood.
- Unoperated cases reaching adulthood usually mild, may present due to associated defects.

Investigation and management
- Echo defines anatomy, degree of obstruction, associated defects. TOE may be required. *Note:*
  - Severity of MS underestimated if coexistent ASD.
  - L-to-R shunt in coexistent ASD exaggerated by MS.
- Surgical repair indicated if significant obstruction.

Cor triatriatum

- Rare, 0.1–0.4% of all congenital heart disease. Associated cardiac defects occur in 70–80% (ASD in 50%).
- A fibromuscular membrane, perforated by ≥1 holes, divides the atrium (nearly always LA) into 2 chambers:
  - Upper chamber receives pulmonary venous return.
  - Lower chamber is the true LA with appendage and MV.

Presentation

- If the holes in the membrane are restrictive → obstructs pulmonary venous blood flow across the membrane into the true LA → supramitral stenosis and presents in childhood.
- If little or no obstruction, may present in adulthood:
  - Incidental finding requiring no treatment.
  - Increasing pulmonary pressures.
  - Atrial fibrillation.
  - Development of mitral regurgitation.

Investigation and management

- CXR:
  - Pulmonary congestion.
  - L atrial appendage not dilated because in low pressure lower chamber.
- Echo—anatomy, functional significance, associated lesions.
- Surgical resection of membrane indicated if causing obstruction to pulmonary venous flow.

Shone syndrome

Obstruction to L ventricular inflow and outflow at multiple levels:
- Supra mitral ring.
- Parachute MV.
- Subvalvular AS.
- Coarctation.

Right ventricular outflow tract obstruction (RVOTO)

Introduction

RVOTO can be due to abnormalities at the following levels:
- Mid RV.
- Infundibulum (as in tetralogy of Fallot).
- PV.
- Supravalvular region.
- Branch ± peripheral PAs.

Pulmonary valvar stenosis

- Usually isolated but occasionally part of a syndrome. 2 main morphological types:
  - Thin, pliable leaflets with dome shape (80–90% cases). May be associated with dilated PA.
  - Dysplastic valve with thickened and immobile leaflets.
- Associated with:
  - Noonan syndrome.
  - Williams syndrome.
  - Alagille syndrome.
- Cardiac associations include ASD.

Symptoms

- Rare in mild-to-moderate stenosis.
- Severe stenosis may present with:
  - Exertional fatigue.
  - Dyspnoea.
  - Chest pain.
  - Atrial arrhythmias.

Physical signs

Key features include:
- RV heave if RVH present.
- Soft delayed P2, ejection systolic murmur at L upper sternal edge.
- Systolic ejection click (if leaflets thin and pliable).
- Cyanosis if severe PS + patent foramen ovale (PFO) or ASD.

Natural and operated history

- Mild PS (PG <30mmHg) rarely deteriorates, does not need long-term follow up after adulthood.
- Moderate PS progresses to need intervention in ~20%.
- After balloon or surgical valvuloplasty most asymptomatic but many have 2° pulmonary regurgitation (PR) → need lifelong follow up.

Investigation

Key points to look for:
- ECG—severe PS: p pulmonale, R axis deviation (RAD), R ventricular hypertrophy (RVH).
- CXR—dilation of main PA, ↓ pulmonary vascular markings if severe PS, Chen's sign = vascular fullness at L base due to preferential flow of turbulent jet into LPA.

- Echo—PV anatomy and severity of PS, RV size and function, associated cardiac abnormalities.
- MRI—quantify RV size and function, identify any pulmonary arterial stenoses.

Intervention

If symptoms, RV dysfunction, moderate–severe PS.

Percutaneous intervention

- Balloon valvuloplasty:
  - Similar long-term results to surgical repair.
  - Suitable for dome-type stenosis.
- Percutaneous valve replacement—new technique, suitable for selected cases, available in limited number of centres.

Surgical intervention

- Valvotomy—subsequent PR more frequent than post-percutaneous intervention.
- Valve replacement.

Supravalvar pulmonary stenosis

- Rarest form of PS, caused by ring of hypertrophic tissue at sinotubular junction of main PA.
- Associated with congenital rubella and Williams syndrome, in which stenosis may occur at multiple levels throughout the pulmonary vasculature.
- Iatrogenic supravalvuar PS may occur post surgery involving main PA (Fallot, arterial switch, and PA banding).
- Examination findings identical to valvar PS except absence of click (suggesting normal pulmonary valve).
- Balloon dilatation rarely successful and surgical correction usually required if severe.

Pulmonary artery stenosis

- Most commonly affects main and lobar arteries.
- Associated with tetralogy of Fallot (post repair), and post-arterial switch repair of TGA. Also seen in Williams syndrome.
- Isolated PA stenosis rare.
- Iatrogenic PA stenosis may occur post systemic to PA shunts.
- 1st-line treatment is balloon dilatation ± stent. However, care must be taken not to compress coronary arteries in the arterial switch patients because of the close relation of the PAs straddling either side of the aorta.

Double-chambered right ventricle

Anomalous muscle bands either → infundibular stenosis or, if lie inferiorly → subinfundibular stenosis and a double-chambered RV.

- Obstruction often mild in childhood but progresses in adulthood as RVH develops.
- Perimembranous VSD usually coexists, may close spontaneously.
- Treatment—surgical resection of obstructing muscle bands.

Ebstein anomaly

Definition

Failure of delamination of the TV leaflets causes apical displacement of the value away from the atrioventricular ring. This leads to:
- Atrialization of the proximal part of the RV → enlarged RA.
- Small functional RV.

📖 See Fig. 7.1.

Incidence

- Rare—1 in 20,000 live births, 0.5% of all congenital heart disease.
- Equal sex incidence.
- Majority of cases are sporadic.
- Associated with maternal ingestion of lithium in the 1st trimester.

Associations

- ASD or PFO in majority.
- 25% Wolf–Parkinson–White syndrome, often with multiple pathways.
- May form part of other complex lesions—tetralogy of Fallot, VSD, PDA, and congenitally corrected TGA.

Natural history

Extremely variable natural history ranging from intrauterine death to presentation in late adulthood. Age at presentation depends on:
- Degree of leaflet displacement.
- Amount of tricuspid regurgitation (TR).
- Functional capacity of RV.
- Associated lesions.

Presenting features in the adult

- Arrhythmia.
- Murmur.
- Progressive cyanosis.
- Paradoxical embolism.
- Heart failure.
- Infective endocarditis.

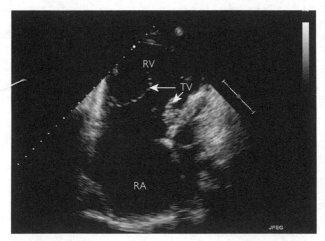

(a)

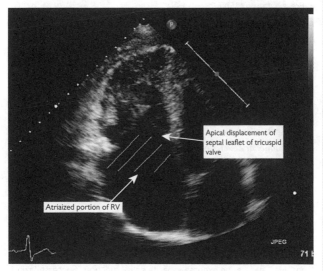

Apical displacement of septal leaflet of tricuspid valve

Atriaized portion of RV

(b)

Fig. 7.1 (a) and (b) Ebstein's anomaly transthoracic echocardiography. Apical 4-chamber views showing tricuspid valve displacement towards the R ventricular apex. The functional RA is very dilated, due to atrialization of part of the RV.

Physical signs

- Cyanosis and clubbing (if R-to-L shunt through ASD or PFO).
- Elevated JVP is a late sign because the TR regurgitant volume is accommodated by the large capacity functional RA.
- Widely split S1 due to ↑ excursion of anterior leaflet.
- S2 variable, may have S3 or S4.
- Tricuspid regurgitant murmur varies from very soft, to loud enough to generate thrill.
- Hepatomegaly, ascites, peripheral oedema—late signs, indicating RV failure.

Investigation

Chest X-ray
Characteristic silhouette and cardiomegaly due to RA enlargement; small aortic knuckle, and oligaemic lung fields.

Electrocardiography
- Superior axis
- RA hypertrophy
- 1st degree heart block (50%)
- RBBB
- Low voltage QRS complexes over right chest leads
- Pre-excitation (25%)

Echocardiography
- Confirms diagnosis—apical displacement of septal ± posterior TV leaflet of >20mm (8mm/m^2).
- Key to planning surgical repair:
  - Anatomy and function of TV.
  - RV size and function.
  - Size of functional RA.
  - Associated structural defects.

MRI
To assess RV dimensions and function.

Cardiopulmonary exercise test
To detect early deterioration in cardiac function.

Management

Non-surgical options
- Symptomatic treatment of heart failure.
- Anticoagulation if atrial arrhythmia present.
- Ablation of accessory pathways.

Surgical options
Timing difficult—aim to repair/replace TV before RV starts to fail. Consider if decreasing exercise capacity or RV function. Successful repair of TV technically difficult and surgery should be carried out only in tertiary centres.

Surgical options are:
- TV replacement.
- TV repair—preferable to replacement; lower mortality and long-term complications.
- Plication of atrialized RV.
- R atrial MAZE procedure.
- Closure of ASD/PFO.
- If RV function poor, combine TV repair with bidirectional Glenn to reduce preload.
- Cardiac transplantation.

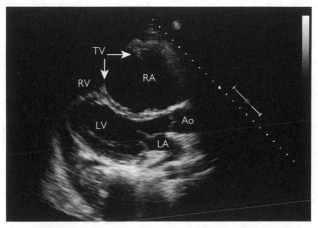

Fig. 7.1 (c) Ebstein's anomaly—transthoracic echocardiography. Parasternal long axis view, showing compression of the LV by the dilated right heart. Ao aorta; LA left atrium; LV left ventricle; RA right atrium; RV right ventricle; TV tricuspid valve.

Septal defects

Atrial septal defects (ASDs)

Introduction

Interatrial communications account for ~10% of congenital heart disease.
Different types of atrial septal defect (ASD) are illustrated in Fig. 8.1.

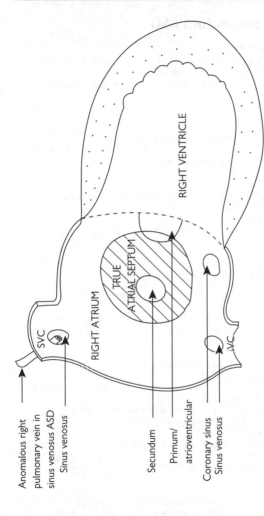

Fig. 8.1 Sites of ASDs. The shaded area delineates the true atrial septum. Sinus venosus and coronary sinus defects are therefore not strictly ASDs although they permit shunting at atrial level.

Ostium secundum ASD

Definition and incidence
- Defect of the oval fossa → direct communication between atrial chambers, allowing shunting of blood.
- Commonest, represents 40% of L-to-R shunts in adults >40 years.
- ♀:♂—2:1.

Associations
- Syndromes:
  - Autosomal dominant familial inheritance.
  - Holt–Oram syndrome—autosomal dominant; skeletal abnormalities and AV conduction defects, due to *TBX5* mutation.
  - Down syndrome.
- Cardiac associations:
  - MV disease—stenosis (MS + ASD known as Lutembacher syndrome), prolapse or regurgitation.
  - PV stenosis.
  - VSD.
  - PDA.
  - CoA.
  - Tetralogy of Fallot.
  - Partial anomalous pulmonary venous connection.

Natural history, presentation, and complications
- Childhood:
  - Isolated ASD usually asymptomatic, murmur may be noted.
  - May present with dyspnoea, recurrent chest infections, sometimes misdiagnosed as asthma.
- Adulthood:
  - May remain undiagnosed for years if symptoms mild because signs subtle and easily missed.
  - Typical presentation—exertional dyspnoea, palpitations, murmur, or dilated R heart on CXR.
- Large ASD not a benign lesion—unoperated, historically only 50% survive to 40 years and 10% beyond 60 years.
- Complications:
  - Atrial fibrillation/flutter—20% by 40 years.
  - R heart failure.
  - Mitral/tricuspid regurgitation.
  - LV dysfunction.
  - PHT:
    —mild (<6 Wood units) common with advancing age.
    —only 10% ASDs develop severe PHT with a R-to-L shunt.
  - Systemic arterial hypertension.
  - Paradoxical embolism.
  - Endocarditis.
- Interactions with other heart disease:
  - LV dysfunction with high LVEDP increases the L-to-R shunt across ASD → ↑ symptoms.

- MV disease:
  —MS and MR both ↑ LA pressure, increasing L-to-R shunt across ASD → ↑ symptoms.
  —severity of MS and MR is underestimated when an ASD coexists, because the LA can decompress through the ASD. If significant MS or MR is missed and the ASD closed, patient may decompensate dramatically.

Physical signs
Points to look for:
- Loud S1, widely split and fixed S2.
- Pulmonary ejection systolic murmur at upper L sternal edge.
- Tricuspid mid-diastolic murmur at lower L sternal edge (due to ↑ flow across TV).
- If R heart failure or PHT:
  - Raised JVP.
  - RV heave at L sternal border.
  - Palpable PA in L 2nd intercostal space.

Investigation
Points to look for:
- ECG—sinus node dysfunction, prolonged P–R interval, RAD, rSr pattern in V1, large P waves.
- CXR—dilated proximal PAs, small aortic knuckle, plethoric lung fields, cardiomegaly (dilatation of RA and RV).
- TTE—dilated, volume overloaded RV, colour flow across interatrial septum, Doppler estimate of PA pressure and any associated lesions.
- Transoesophageal echocardiogram—define number, site, size, and rims of ASD, identify PVs.
- Cardiac catheterization—calculation of pulmonary vascular resistance and assessment of coexistent congenital or acquired cardiac pathology e.g. coronary artery disease.

ASD repair
Indications for closure of ASD
- R heart volume overload.
- L-to-R shunt ≥1.5:1 and ASD ≥10mm in diameter.
- Prevention of recurrent paradoxical embolism.
- Benefits of closure of haemodynamically significant ASD are improved:
  - Survival.
  - Functional class.
  - Exercise tolerance.
  - Reduction of risk of heart failure.

Contraindications to ASD closure
- Significant pulmonary vascular disease.
- Severe LV dysfunction.
- Significant MV disease.

Methods of closure

- Percutaneous closure may be performed for isolated secundum ASD if:
  - <4cm diameter.
  - Anatomically away from AV valves, pulmonary and caval veins.
  - Normal pulmonary venous drainage.
- Risk—1–2% major complication.
- Antiplatelet therapy recommended for 3–6 months post-closure.
- Surgical repair ± Maze procedure. Mortality similar to device closure, but postoperative AF common and recovery longer.

Prognosis post ASD repair

- Repair by 20 years—normal life expectancy, late complications unlikely.
- Repair after 25 years—late atrial arrhythmia may occur.
- Repair after 40 years—functional capacity improved, longevity may be less than normal population but better than if unrepaired.

Ostium primum ASD

Definition
- The septum primum is deficient (📖 see Fig. 8.1, p.95).
- The primum ASD is the atrial component of an AVSD (📖 see Chapter 8c, Atrioventricular septal defects (AVSDs), pp.109–112)

Sinus venosus ASD

Definition and incidence
- SVC type more common than IVC type.
- A defect of infolding of the atrial wall → SVC connects to both atria, creating an interatrial communication, outside the atrial septum—not a 'true' defect of the atrial septum. R-sided partial anomalous venous drainage is an integral part of the defect.
- Incidence: 2–3% of ASDs, ♀ = ♂.

Associations
- Anomalous pulmonary venous drainage.
- Ectopic atrial pacemaker (defect in area of SA node).

Presentation
As for secundum ASD.

Cautions:
- May not be seen using TTE. TOE needed to define the defect and associated anomalous pulmonary venous drainage.
- Unsuitable for percutaneous closure:
  - No superior rim to the defect.
  - Anomalous pulmonary venous drainage.

Coronary sinus defect

- Rare.
- Defect is at the entry site of the coronary sinus to the LA.
- Mildest form = simple fenestration in atrial wall by the opening of the coronary sinus.
- Unroofed coronary sinus = variation in which the roof separating the coronary sinus from the LA is absent. A persistent LSVC draining to the coronary sinus usually coexists, resulting in a R-to-L shunt and cyanosis.

Patent foramen ovale

Definition and incidence
- PFO is a normal variant found in up to 30% of the population.
- Results from failure of fusion of the valve of the foramen ovale with the septum after birth when the LA pressure exceeds that of the RA—there is no deficiency of atrial septal tissue.

Presentation
- Incidental finding.
- Paradoxical embolism or embolism of thrombus *in situ:*
  - Cryptogenic stroke in young adults.
  - Neurological decompression sickness following diving.
- Migraine with aura may be associated with PFO.

Physical signs and investigations
- Signs—none, except from any previous neurological deficit.
- ECG, CXR, and TTE are normal.
- Contrast echo:
  - PFO is likely if, with Valsalva, bubbles appear in the LA within 5 heart beats.
  - Should only be performed if there is a management plan in the event of a PFO being found—knowledge of the existence of a PFO for which there is no indication for closure may cause unnecessary anxiety.

Indications for closure of PFO
- Patients with previous embolic stroke, PFO, and risk factors for venous thrombosis appear to be protected against further events by device closure.
- Careful risk assessment must be made in all patients with an embolic stroke prior to device closure because if multiple risk factors (e.g. smoking, hypertension, diabetes, hyperlipidaemia, or proven atherosclerotic disease) or factors for L-sided intracardiac thrombosis (e.g. AF, MV disease with a dilated LA) are present, device closure is unlikely to reduce further events.
- Current research is investigating whether PFO closure will benefit migraine sufferers.
- Percutaneous closure is performed as for secundum ASDs. Antiplatelet or anticoagulant therapy is recommended for 6 months post-procedure. However, aspirin should be continued long term if arterial thromboembolism was a possible case for the neurological event.

Ventricular septal defects (VSDs)

Definition and incidence

- Common—3 per 1000 live births. ♀ = ♂.
- Due to developmental failure of 1 of the ventricular septal components—inlet septum, muscular trabeculated septum, outlet septum, or perimembranous septum.
- VSDs are classified by their location within the septum and by their borders viewed from the RV (📖 see Fig. 8.2).
  - Muscular.
  - Perimembranous VSD (pVSD)—commonest type in Europe and N America.
  - Doubly committed subarterial—only ~5% of European and N American VSDs, up to 30% of Asian VSDs.

See larger texts for more detail.

Cardiac associations

Occurs as:
- Isolated defect.
- In association with other lesions e.g. coarctation.
- As integral part of e.g. tetralogy of Fallot.

Presentation

Depends on size and haemodynamic effects of VSD.
- Children:
  - Small defects—often asymptomatic. Spontaneous closure of perimembranous or small muscular VSD common.
  - Moderate or large VSD—may present with failure to thrive and congestive heart failure.
- Adults:
  - Unoperated restrictive VSDs usually asymptomatic.
  - Survivors of large unoperated VSDs are likely to have developed pulmonary vascular disease (Eisenmenger syndrome).
- AR may develop in perimembranous and doubly-committed subarterial VSDs.
- Atrial fibrillation is a late complication, associated with LA and LV dilation and dysfunction

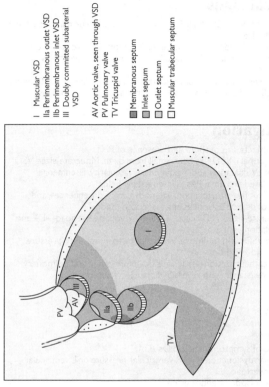

I   Muscular VSD
IIa Perimembranous outlet VSD
IIb Perimembranous inlet VSD
III Doubly committed subarterial
    VSD

AV Aortic valve, seen through VSD
PV Pulmonary valve
TV Tricuspid valve

■ Membranous septum
■ Inlet septum
□ Outlet septum
□ Muscular trabecular septum

Fig. 8.2 (🕮 See also Plate 3) Schematic representation to show the sites of different types of VSDs.
The heart is in cross section, viewed from the R ventricular aspect.

Physical signs

- Small restrictive VSD—high-frequency pansystolic murmur loudest at
  L sternal edge,
- Moderate-to-large non-restrictive VSD—displaced cardiac apex,
  pansystolic murmur, apical diastolic murmur and S3 from ↑ flow
  through the MV
- Eisenmenger VSD—cyanosis, clubbing, RV heave, palpable and loud P2,
  S4, systolic and diastolic murmurs (pulmonary dilatation and PR).

Investigation

- ECG—reflects size of shunt and presence of PHT.
- CXR—normal if VSD has been small from birth. Moderate-sized VSD
  results in LV dilatation and ↑ pulmonary vascularity. Eisenmenger
  VSD—dilated proximal PAs, oligaemic lung fields.
- Echo—identifies size, location, haemodynamic consequences, and
  number of defects as well as any associated lesions.
  - Moderate-sized VSDs cause LA and LV volume overload—LA and
    LV dilation.
  - Large VSDs with pulmonary vascular disease cause RV pressure
    overload—RVH.
- Cardiac catheterization—calculate size of the shunt and pulmonary
  vascular resistance with reversibility studies if appropriate.

Repair

Indications

- Presence of symptoms and Qp:Qs >2:1.
- Ventricular dysfunction with R ventricular pressure or L ventricular
  volume overload.
- Previous episode of endocarditis.
- AR due to aortic valve prolapse into perimembranous or doubly
  committed subarterial VSDs.

Surgical repair

- The conducting tissue is vulnerable in perimembranous defects. R bundle
  branch block very common after repair of pVSD. Postoperative transient
  heart block may occur; if persists, permanent pacemaker insertion
  recommended because of risk of late sudden death.
- Transatrial repair reduces risk of late RV tachycardia and dysfunction
  that may occur after transventricular approach.
- Long-term postoperative survival dependent on PHT, LV dysfunction
  and complications such AR and endocarditis.

Percutaneous closure

Selected muscular and pVSDs may be device closed in specialist centres.
Particular care is required for the assessment and closure of pVSDs to
avoid heart block and damage to the aortic valve.

Atrioventricular septal defects (AVSDs)

Definition

- Key feature = common atrioventricular (AV) junction and AV valve ring.
- The atrial component of an AVSD = ostium primum ASD.
- The normal 'off-setting' of the AV valves is absent. Apical 4-chamber echo:
  - Normal—tricuspid valve lies further towards the apex than the MV.
  - AVSD—both AV valves lie at the same level.
- The AV valves are not true MV and TVs; they are termed L and R AV valves. They share 5 leaflets between them and are potentially regurgitant.
- The aorta is 'unwedged' from its normal position between the AV valves → long LV outflow tract with risk of obstruction.

Note: AVSD was previously termed endocardial cushion defect or atrioventricular canal

There are 2 types of AVSD (Fig. 8.3)
- *Partial AVSD*—R and L AV valves have separate orifices and VSD is usually small or absent. >90% occur in non-Down patients.
- *Complete AVSD*—common AV valve and valve orifice with large VSD. >75% occur in Down patients.

Associations

- Strongly associated with trisomy 21, especially complete AVSD.
- May occur with tetralogy of Fallot and double-outlet RV.

Incidence and recurrence

- ♀ = ♂.
- Recurrence risk is high—up to 10% if the mother is affected.

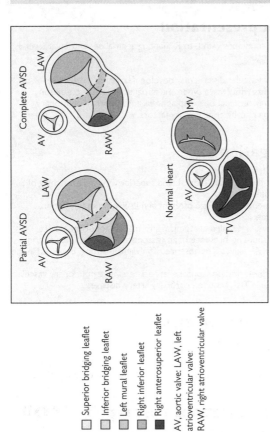

☐ Superior bridging leaflet
☐ Inferior bridging leaflet
☐ Left mural leaflet
☐ Right inferior leaflet
☐ Right anterosuperior leaflet

AV, aortic valve; LAW, left
atrioventricular valve;
RAW, right atrioventricular valve

Fig. 8.3. (☐ See also Plate 4) Schematic representation of the atrioventricular junction in AVSD. Short axis view seen from the atrial aspect.. In both forms of AVSD there is a common atrioventricular valve ring guarded by 5 valve leaflets. In the partial defect the superior and inferior bridging leaflets fuse to create 2 separate valve orifices. This fusion does not occur in complete AVSD, so there is a common valve orifice

Clinical presentation

As for other conditions with L-to-R shunting at atrial or ventricular level, ±:
- AV valve regurgitation.
- LVOTO.
- Pulmonary vascular disease may develop if large non restrictive VSD. Patients with Down syndrome at particular risk—co-existing upper airway obstruction, sleep apnoea, and abnormal pulmonary parenchyma may be contributory factors.

Investigation

Points to look for:
- ECG—1st-degree heart block, L and superior QRS axis, notching of S waves in inferior leads.
- CXR—depends on the size of shunt and LAV valve regurgitation; cardiomegaly
- TTE—provides detailed anatomical information about the defect, degree of shunting, presence of any associated LVOTO, function and anatomy of AV valves. The absence of valvar 'off-setting' is viewed in the 4-chamber view.
- Cardiac catheterization—preoperative assessment: pulmonary vascular resistance, LVOTO, acquired coronary artery disease.

Surgical management

- *Partial AVSD*—pericardial patch closure of primum ASD with repair of left AV valve.
- *Complete AVSD*—ASD and VSD repair with AV valve reconstruction. Surgical repair should not be performed if severe irreversible PHT.

Late complications post repair of AVSD

- Recurrent AV regurgitation.
- Residual ASD or VSD.
- Residual or recurrent LVOTO.
- Complete heart block.
- Atrial arrhythmia.
- Endocarditis.

All patients require long-term follow-up because of the risk of LAV valve regurgitation, LVOTO, atrial arrhythmias, or conduction abnormalities.

The Eisenmenger syndrome

Introduction

Large communication between the systemic and pulmonary circulations at atrial, ventricular, or arterial level:
→ high pulmonary blood flow (L-to-R shunt);
→ development of high pulmonary vascular resistance;
→ reversed or bidirectional shunt (R-to-L shunt);
→ cyanosis with PHT at systemic level.
• Incidence is reducing—surgery in infancy should prevent the Eisenmenger syndrome developing in most cases.
• One of the most vulnerable conditions to iatrogenic complications.

Natural history

Exercise tolerance usually significantly limited, but survival into the 5th decade is common, and is reported into the 8th decade, much better than for other forms of pulmonary arterial hypertension.

Markers of poor prognosis / disease progression include:
• Complex anatomy and physiology.
• Decline in functional class.
• Heart failure.
• Arrhythmia.
• Rising serum uric acid.

Complications and extra-cardiac manifestations

📖 see Cyanosis, pp.57–62.

Physical signs

• Cyanosis, clubbing.
• RV heave.
• Loud P2.
• May have pulmonary ejection click and PR.
• No murmur from causative communication e.g. VSD, since equal pressures on either side.
• Discriminatory signs:
  • VSD—single S2.
  • ASD—often fixed split S2.
  • PDA—normally split S2; differential cyanosis—pink fingers, blue toes.

Investigations

Points to look for:
- ECG—p pulmonale, RVH.
- CXR—dilated proximal PAs, oligaemic lung fields.
- Echo—site of shunt, estimation of pulmonary arterial pressure, and ventricular function.
- CPE—caution, maximal exercise testing may induce potentially fatal syncope. 6-min walk may be better measure of exercise capacity.
- Multislice CT scanning to show:
  - Hypertensive pulmonary vasculature.
  - Collateral vessels.
  - *In situ* pulmonary thrombus.
  - PA aneurysms.
  - Site of any pulmonary haemorrhage.
- Cardiac catheterization: unnecessary and potentially dangerous. Only indication is if suspect reversibility of the high pulmonary vascular resistance: if confirmed, corrective surgery may be possible. This situation is rarely encountered in the adult population.

Management

- General measures—📖 see Cyanosis, pp.57–62.
- Selective pulmonary vasodilators may have a role. Referral to specialist centre required.
- Surgical repair of causative lesion not possible.
- Heart–lung transplantation limited by complex anatomy and donor availability.

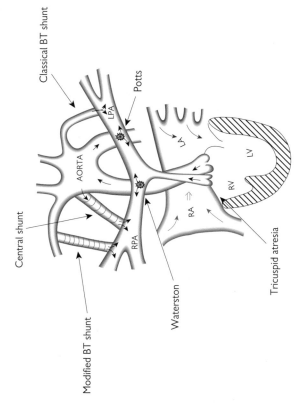

Plate 1 Types of systemic–pulmonary arterial shunts (tricuspid atresia). (□ See also Fig. 5.2, p.54)

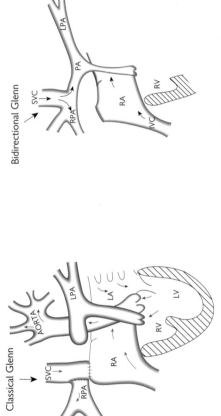

Plate 2 Systemic venous to pulmonary arterial shunts—the Glenn anastomosis. (See also Fig. 5.3, p.55)

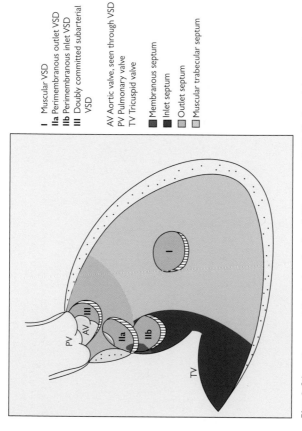

I   Muscular VSD
IIa Perimembranous outlet VSD
IIb Perimembranous inlet VSD
III Doubly committed subarterial VSD

AV Aortic valve, seen through VSD
PV Pulmonary valve
TV Tricuspid valve

■ Membranous septum
■ Inlet septum
□ Outlet septum
□ Muscular trabecular septum

Plate 3 Schematic representation to show the sites of different types of VSDs. The heart is in cross section, viewed from the R ventricular aspect. (🔲 See also Fig. 8.2, p.107)

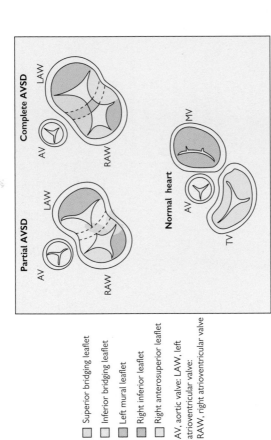

Plate 4 Schematic representation of the atrioventricular junction in AVSD. Short axis view seen from the atrial aspect. In both forms of AVSD there is a common atrioventricular valve ring guarded by 5 valve leaflets. In the partial defect the superior and inferior bridging leaflets fuse to create 2 separate valve orifices. This fusion does not occur in complete AVSD, so there is a common valve orifice. (▢ See also Fig. 8.3, p.111)

☐ Superior bridging leaflet
☐ Inferior bridging leaflet
☐ Left mural leaflet
☐ Right inferior leaflet
☐ Right anterosuperior leaflet

AV, aortic valve; LAW, left atrioventricular valve;
RAW, right atrioventricular valve

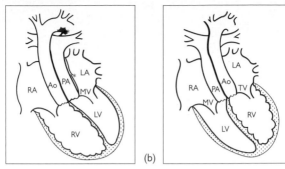

Plate 5 Transposition complexes. (a) Schematic representation of complete TGA (ventriculoarterial discordance). (b) Schematic representation of ccTGA (atrio ventricular and ventriculoarterial discordance). Ao aorta; LA left atrium; LV left ventricle; PA pulmonary artery; MV mitral valve; RA right atrium; RV right ventricle; TV tricuspid valve; **patent foramen ovale; *patent arterial duct. (📖 See also Fig. 12.1, p.145)

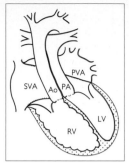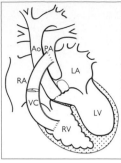

(a) (b)

Plate 6 Surgical approaches to complete TGA. (a) Schematic representation of interatrial repair (Senning or Mustard operation). (b) Schematic representation of Rastelli operation. Ao aorta; LA left atrium; LV left ventricle; PA pulmonary artery; RA right atrium; RV right ventricle; VC valved conduit. Ao aorta; LV left ventricle; PA pulmonary artery; PVA pulmonary venous atrium; RV right ventricle; SVA systemic venous atrium. (📖 See also Fig. 12.2, p.149)

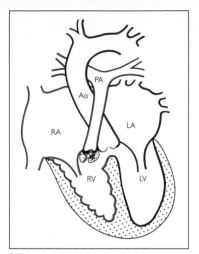

Plate 7 Schematic representation of unoperated tetralogy of Fallot. * deviation of outlet septum, Ao aorta; LA left atrium; LV left ventricle; PA pulmonary artery; RA right atrium; RV right ventricle. (📖 See also Fig. 13.1, p.161)

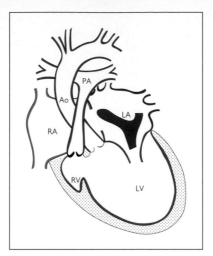

Plate 8 Schematic representation of tricuspid atresia. Systemic venous blood leaves the RA via an atrial septal defect and mixes with pulmonary venous blood in the LA. The LV thus supports both the systemic and pulmonary circulations and the patient is cyanosed. The rudimentary RV does not play a functional role. Ao aorta; LA left atrium; LV left ventricle; PA pulmonary artery; RA right atrium; RV right ventricle. (□ See also Fig. 14.1, p.173)

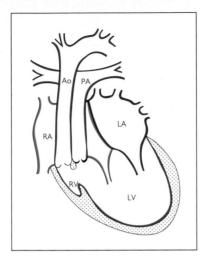

Plate 9 Schematic representation of double inlet LV with VA discordance. Both atria connect to the LV via the tricuspid and mitral valves, so that systemic and pulmonary venous blood mix in the LV and the patient is cyanosed. The LV supports both the systemic and pulmonary circulations. The aorta arises from the rudimentary RV via the VSD. If the VSD is restrictive, it creates obstruction to systemic blood flow. Ao aorta; LA left atrium; LV left ventricle; PA pulmonary artery; RA right atrium; RV right ventricle; VA ventriculoarterial; VSD ventricular septal defect. (📖 See also Fig. 14.2, p.173)

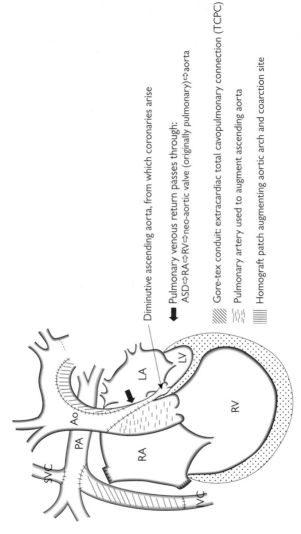

Diminutive ascending aorta, from which coronaries arise

Pulmonary venous return passes through:
ASD⇨RA⇨RV⇨neo-aortic valve (originally pulmonary)⇨aorta

Gore-tex conduit: extracardiac total cavopulmonary connection (TCPC)

Pulmonary artery used to augment ascending aorta

Homograft patch augmenting aortic arch and coarction site

Plate 10 Schematic representation of hypoplastic left heart following Stage 3 Fontan palliation. Ao aorta; IVC inferior vena cava; LA left atrium; LV left ventricle; PA pulmonary artery; RA right atrium; RV right ventricle; SVC superior vena cava. (🖳 See also Fig. 14.8, p.187)

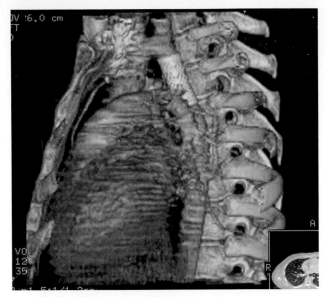

Plate 11 Multislice CT scan to show coarctation stent.

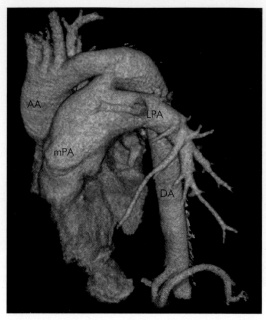

Plate 12 Eisenmenger PDA. 3D reconstruction from multi-slice CT scan demonstrating a PDA (arrow) in a 36-year-old woman with Eisenmenger syndrome. AA ascending aorta; DA descending aorta; LPA and mPA left and main pulmonary artery (📖 See Fig. 2.19, p.31).

Aortic lesions

Coarctation of the aorta (CoA)

📖 See Fig. 10.1.

Definition and incidence

- Narrowing of aorta, usually just distal to L subclavian artery.
- Considerable variation in anatomy and severity, from mild, localized obstruction to interruption or hypoplasia of the arch.
- Incidence 1:12 000 live births.
- ♂ to ♀ ratio of 3:1.

Associations

- Bicuspid aortic valve present in up to 80%.
- VSD.
- PDA.
- MV abnormalities.
- Turner syndrome.
- Aneurysm of the circle of Willis.

Natural history

- Most present acutely in infancy; unoperated outlook is poor.
- Unoperated survival beyond infancy occurs if:
  - CoA coarctation is mild, *or*
  - Adequate collateral circulation exists.
- Majority of unoperated survivors die by 50 years from premature coronary disease, stroke, or aortic dissection.

Presentation

In infancy:

- L ventricular heart failure.
- Systolic murmur.
- Reduced femoral pulses with radio femoral delay.
- Upper body hypertension.
- BP gradient between R upper and lower extremities.

In adulthood:

- Hypertension
- During investigation for bicuspid aortic valve disease.
- Less commonly:
  - Leg claudication.
  - Heart failure.
  - Cerebral haemorrhage.

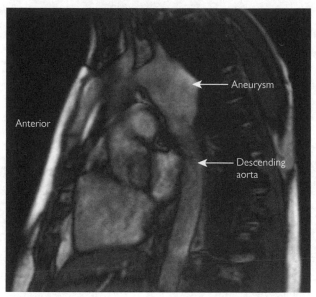

Fig. 10.1 Aneurysm post-patch repair of CoA. Sagittal section view of an MRI scan of a 25-year-old ♂ who underwent Dacron patch repair of a coarctation age 3 months. He developed an aneurysm at the site of repair that expanded on serial MRI studies. He therefore underwent surgical repair of the aneurysm.

Physical signs

Points to look for:
- R brachial BP higher than L if L subclavian artery involved in:
  - Native CoA.
  - CoA repair.
  - → *BP should be measured in right arm for all CoA.*
- Radiofemoral delay.
- Aortic ejection murmur and ejection click from bicuspid aortic valve.
- Ejection murmur over back from CoA.
- Palpable collaterals over back.
- Hypertensive retinopathy.

Investigations

Points to look for:
- CXR—Fig. 10.2, p.121, shows features of unoperated CoA.
- ECG—LVH.
- Echocardiography:
  - LVH.
  - Supra sternal Doppler—↑ velocity in DA (peak gradient >20mmHg and diastolic tail).
  - Associated lesions
- MRI (📖 see Fig. 10.1).
  - Haemodynamic data.
  - 2- and 3D images of site, collaterals, and related vessels

Management

- Surgical repair preferred in infants and children, with a risk of <1%. Initial anatomy and surgical approach determines risk of late complication. Patch repair associated with late aneurysm formation.
- Transcatheter balloon dilatation and stenting is an alternative to surgery in selected:
  - Adults and older children.
  - Operated patients with residual CoA.
  - The procedure carries a risk of aortic dissection and aneurysm formation; its practice should be confined to specialist centres.

Late outcome and follow-up

Late survival is 92% for patients repaired in infancy, 15-year survival is only 50% for those repaired at age >40 years.

Late complications are associated with:
- Arterial hypertension.
- Recoarctation or residual stenosis.
- Aneurysm formation (Dacron patch).
- Progression of associated lesions.

Lifelong follow up required:
- Clinical examination every 1–3 years—BP of all extremities, peripheral pulses.
- ECG.
- MRI (or CT) every 5 years.

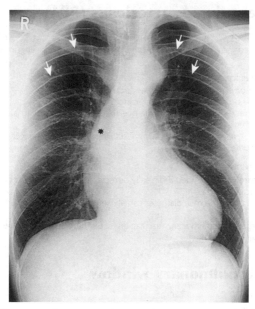

Fig. 10.2 Chest radiograph of an 18-year-old man with unoperated coarctation of the aorta and bicuspid aortic valve. There is bilateral rib notching (arrows), a dilated ascending aorta (*), and a prominent deformed aortic knuckle.

1 Kirklin JW, Barratt-Boyes BG (1993). *Cardiac surgery*, 2nd edn. New York: Churchill Livingstone Inc.

Patent ductus arteriosus (PDA)

Definition
PDA = connection between AA and proximal LPA, persisting from fetal life.

Consequences
Depend on size of shunt. Risk of endocarditis very small.
- Small—no haemodynamic significance.
- Moderate—late L heart volume overload, LV dysfunction, atrial arrhythmia.
- Large—may result in pulmonary vascular disease (Eisenmenger syndrome, 📖 see p.113).

Management
- Closure recommended if clinically detectable i.e. continuous murmur in L subclavian area.
- Ducts up to 14mm in diameter usually suitable for transcatheter closure.
- In large ducts, pulmonary vascular disease should be excluded before repair is undertaken.

Aortopulmonary window

Definition
- Rare; direct communication between adjacent portions of proximal AA and PA.
- Communication usually large; physiological consequences the same as PDA.
- Rare patients surviving unoperated into adulthood likely to have developed the Eisenmenger reaction.
- Long-term postoperative survival is good if there was low pulmonary vascular resistance at repair.

Common arterial trunk/truncus arteriosus

Definition
A single great artery arises from the heart and gives rise to the coronary arteries, aorta, and PAs. There is a semilunar 'truncal' valve that has ≥3 leaflets, and a subtruncal VSD. It may coexist with interrupted aortic arch, CoA, coronary anomalies and DiGeorge syndrome.

Management and late complications
The majority undergo surgery within the 1st year of life.
- Closure of the VSD.
- Detachment of the PA from the common trunk.
- Placement of a valved R ventricular-to-pulmonary artery conduit.
- The truncal valve function as the aortic valve.

20-year survival is >80% in patients <1 year at operation. Late complications are related to:
- Truncal (aortic) regurgitation.
- Truncal (aortic root) dilatation.
- Ventricular dysfunction.
- Conduit stenosis or regurgitation (multiple replacements).
- Myocardial ischemia (coronary abnormalities).
- Arrhythmia.

Follow up
Annual follow up is recommended and should include:
- ECG—arrhythmia, ventricular hypertrophy.
- Echocardiography—truncal valve function, conduit function, aortic root dimension, ventricular function, branch pulmonary artery stenosis.

Periodically or on specific indication or suspicion:
- Holter monitoring—suspected arrhythmia.
- MRI—poor echocardiographic window, pre-intervention.
- Exercise testing—functional capacity, suspected ischemia, pre-interventional.

Marfan syndrome

Definition
- Autosomal dominant defect of connective tissue due to mutations in the *fibrillin-1 (FBN1)* gene.
- It is a multi-organ disease; the diagnosis is based on clinical findings.[1]
- There is an overlap with other connective tissue disorders like Loeys–Dietz syndrome—a particularly aggressive disease strongly associated with aortic aneurysm.
- Cardiovascular diagnostic criteria include:
  - *Major:*
    - —aortic root dilatation.
    - —dissection of AA.
  - *Minor:*
    - —MV prolapse and/or calcification.
    - —dilatation of the PA.
    - —dilatation or dissection of the DA.

Management
All patients should be recommended:
- Beta-blocker therapy.
- Avoidance of more than mild static and moderate dynamic exercise and sports with the risk of bodily collision.

Surgery should be considered in patients with:
- Aortic root dimension >50–55mm.
- Aortic root dimension >40–45mm in high-risk situations:
  - Patients planning pregnancy.
  - Family history of premature aortic dissection and rupture.
  - Rapid annual aortic root growth (>5%).
  - Patients with Loeys–Dietz syndrome.

A valve-sparing procedure should be encouraged.

Follow up
Annual cardiac follow up is mandatory in all Marfan patients.

Echocardiography
- Aortic root dimensions.
- Ascending or abdominal aortic dissection.
- Aortic valve regurgitation.
- L ventricular size and function.
- MV prolapse/regurgitation.

MRI
- Complete aortic assessment.
- Follow-up of chronic dissection.

The angiotensin II receptor antagonist, losartan, acting as a TGFβ antagonist, has been shown to act to prevent disease progression in animal models of Marfan syndrome. There are ongoing trials in humans.

1 De Paepe A, Devereux RB, Dietz HC, *et al.* (1996). Revised diagnostic criteria for the Marfan syndrome. *Am J Med Genet* **62**(4), 417–26.

Venous anomalies

Anomalies of systemic venous drainage

Introduction

Commonly seen as part of complex disorder.

Superior vena cava (SVC) anomalies

Persistent LSVC (see Fig. 11.1)

Occurs due to failure of the LSVC to obliterate during embryogenesis.
- Usually drains into RA via CS.
- RSVC usually present too.
- Present in:
  - 0.3% general population.
  - 3% of all patients with congenital heart disease.
  - 15% of patients with tetralogy of Fallot.
- No haemodynamic significance but may cause difficulty during transvenous pacing.
- Diagnosis:
  - Echo—dilated CS.
  - CXR—LSVC may be visible.

LSVC connection to LA

- Rare.
- LSVC connects directly to LA.
- Associated with isomerism.
- Obligatory R-to-L shunt causes cyanosis.
- Diagnosis made by L-arm bubble contrast echo. NB diagnosis will be missed if bubble contrast echo performed with R-arm injection

Absent RSVC

- Rare.
- Associated with:
  - Complete heart block.
  - Sinus node dysfunction.
  - Atrial fibrillation.

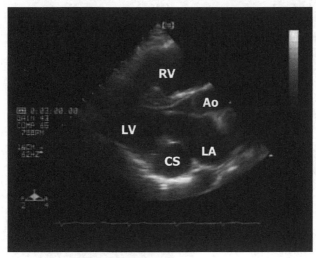

Fig. 11.1 Persistent LSVC draining to coronary sinus. 2D TTE; parasternal long axis view to show CS dilated due to receiving blood from a persistent LSVC. Ao aorta; CS coronary sinus; LA left atrium; LV left ventricle; RV right ventricle.

Inferior vena cava (IVC) anomalies

Azygous continuation of IVC
- Absent infrahepatic portion of IVC.
- Continues as azygous vein.
- Hepatic veins drain directly into RA.
- Present in 0.6% of congenital heart disease.
- Associated with complex lesions, particularly L-atrial isomerism.
- Diagnosis—CXR (absence of IVC at R cardiophrenic border and dilated azygous vein).
  - Ultrasound or other non-invasive imaging.

Anomalies of pulmonary venous drainage

Total anomalous pulmonary venous drainage (TAPVD)

Definition

- All 4 pulmonary veins drain into R heart.
- Either drain directly into RA or via a common vein into a systemic vein:
  - *Supracardiac course* draining to SVC, azygous or innominate vein.
  - *Cardiac course* draining either into RA, CS, or persistent LSVC.
  - *Infradiaphragmatic course* draining to portal vein or IVC.
- Strongest predictor of poor outcome is pulmonary venous obstruction.

Incidence and associations

- 1 in 17 000 live births.
- Obligatory R-to-L shunt, usually ASD.
- PDA.
- May coexist with complex cyanotic lesions and R atrial isomerism.

Natural and operated history

- 98 % present in infancy with dyspnoea, cyanosis, failure to thrive.
- Symptoms due to obstruction of pulmonary venous drainage.

Operated course

- Early deaths virtually confined to those with obstructed pulmonary venous drainage.
- Excellent prognosis in surgical survivors.
- May develop obstruction of redirected pulmonary venous pathway in the growing child.
- Once fully grown, patients with no residual obstruction or associated lesions may be discharged from follow up.

Unoperated course

- Rarely reach adulthood (only if large ASD and unobstructed pulmonary venous drainage).
- Cyanosis.
- Pulmonary vascular disease.
- R heart failure.
- Atrial arrhythmias.

Partial anomalous pulmonary venous drainage (PAPVD)

Definition
- ≥1 PVs drain into R heart.
- R upper or R middle PV to SVC or RA in 90% of cases.

Associations
ASD—10–15% of all ASDs; 80–90% of sinus venosus ASDs.

Natural history and presentation
- May present in adult life, as L-to-R shunt at atrial level.
- Suspect if unexplained R heart dilatation and intact intra atrial septum.
- Symptoms same as ASD and relate to magnitude of L-to-R shunt:
  - Exertional dyspnoea.
  - Atrial arrhythmias.
  - R heart failure.
  - PHT.

Diagnosis
- ECG—right bundle branch block (RBBB).
- CXR—may show abnormally draining vein.
- TTE—dilated R heart, difficult to identify PVs in adults.
- TOE—required to identify all 4 PVs.
- MRI—identifies anomalous PVs draining to systemic veins.

Intervention
- Indications for surgical repair same as for ASD.
- Excellent long-term outcome following surgical repair.
- Long-term complications of repair include:
  - Obstruction of re-implanted PV.
  - Atrial arrhythmias.
  - Obstruction of systemic venous return (very rare).

Scimitar syndrome

📖 See Fig. 11.2.
- Rare, familial syndrome affecting 1–3/100 000 live births.
- Definition:
  - Part or all of the RPVs drain to the IVC below the diaphragm.
  - Arterial supply of affected R lung (usually lower lobe) from DA.
  - Affected lung lobes usually hypoplastic.
- Associated cardiac lesions in 25% cases (ASD, VSD, PDA, coarctation, Fallot)

Presentation
- L-to-R shunt.
- Severe forms associated with other lesions present in infancy; high mortality.
- May present with bronchiectasis, recurrent chest infections and haemoptysis in affected lobes.
- As incidental CXR finding.

Diagnosis
- CXR—shows anomalous PV (said to resemble a Turkish sword—'a Scimitar'). 📖 See Fig. 11.3.
- MRI—demonstrates abnormal venous drainage and arterial supply.

Management
- Intervention rarely required in adults.
- Lobectomy or pneumonectomy may be indicated if recurrent chest infections, haemoptysis, or marked hypoplasia.

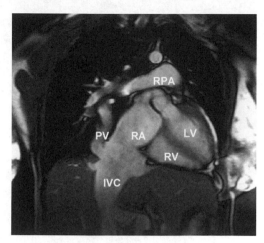

Fig. 11.2. Scimitar syndrome. Coronal section MRI scan demonstrating the anomalous RPV (that creates the 'scimitar' shape on the chest radiograph) draining to the IVC. IVC inferior vena cava; LV left ventricle; PV pulmonary vein; RA right atrium; RPA right pulmonary artery; RV right ventricle.

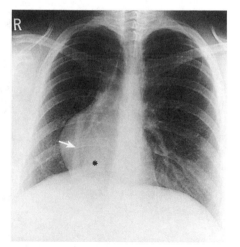

Fig. 11.3. Chest radiograph of a 25-year-old woman with Scimitar syndrome. The heart is shifted into the R hemithorax because the R lung is small. The scimitar shadow (arrow) is produced by the anomalous descending venous channel which drains into the dilated IVC (*).

Transposition complexes

Complete transposition of the great arteries (TGA)

Introduction

There are 2 types of TGA (📖 see Fig. 12.1):

1. Complete TGA

Described as atrioventricular (AV) concordance, ventriculoarterial (VA) discordance. Previously also known as D-TGA.

Once the arterial duct and foramen ovale have closed, incompatible with life without intervention, because there is complete separation of the systemic and pulmonary circulations:

• Deoxygenated blood from the systemic veins recirculates to the aorta.
• Oxygenated blood from the pulmonary veins recirculates to the pulmonary artery.

2. Congenitally corrected TGA (ccTGA)

Described as AV and VA discordance. Previously known as L-TGA.

ccTGA is congenitally physiologically 'corrected' since:

• Deoxygenated systemic venous blood reaches the pulmonary artery, albeit via the morphological LV.
• Oxygenated pulmonary venous blood reaches the aorta, but via the morphological RV.

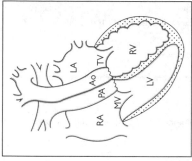

(a)

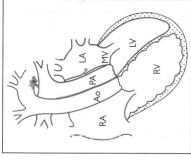

(b)

Fig. 12.1 (See also Plate 5) Transposition complexes. (a) Schematic representation of complete TGA (ventriculoarterial discordance). (b) Schematic representation of ccTGA (atrioventricular and ventriculoarterial discordance). Ao aorta; LA left atrium; LV left ventricle; PA pulmonary artery; MV mitral valve; RA right atrium; RV right ventricle; TV tricuspid valve; *patent foramen ovale; **patent arterial duct.

Complete TGA

AV concordance, VA discordance; 📖 see Fig. 12.1(a), p.145.

Introduction
- 5% of all congenital heart disease.
- ♂:♀ ratio = 4:1.
- 📖 see Introduction, p.4 for description of connections and physiology.

Cardiac associations
- 40–50% VSD.
- Up to 25% LVOTO (subpulmonary stenosis) or pulmonary valvar stenosis.
- 5% CoA.

Natural (unoperated) history
- TGA and intact interventricular septum—only about 10% survive beyond the 1st year of life, because of failure of mixing of blood. Those that do survive have mixing at the level of the atria or duct.
- TGA with VSD and PS—mixing of oxygenated and deoxygenated blood occurs at ventricular level, and excessive pulmonary blood flow is prevented, resulting in a 'balanced' cyanotic circulation that may allow survival into adulthood.

Operated history
3 main surgical approaches to repair; the approach taken influences the long term outcome:[1]
- Interatrial repair—Mustard or Senning operation.
- Arterial switch operation.
- Rastelli operation.

1 Warnes CA (2006). Transposition of the great arteries. *Circulation* **114**(24), 2699–709.

Interatrial repair—Mustard or Senning operation

📖 See Fig. 12.2(a)

The atrial septum is excised and a saddle-shaped patch ('baffle') is placed to direct pulmonary venous blood into the RA and RV and thence to the aorta. Systemic venous blood is directed into the LA, LV, and into the PA. The RV (and TV) therefore continue to support the systemic circulation.

Rarely performed now; superseded by the arterial switch operation since the late 1980s (📖 see Arterial switch operation, p.150). However, there are many adult survivors of the approach who face inevitable late complications.

Complications of Mustard/Senning operations

- Arrhythmia—very common due to extensive atrial surgery (📖 see also Chapter, 16, p.204):
  - Bradycardia and sinus node dysfunction is often progressive.
  - Tachycardia—*atrial flutter* occurs in up to 50% of patients, commoner with advancing age. Poorly tolerated and may conduct 1:1. It is a likely cause of sudden death. *Urgent DC conversion is required. Pharmocological attempts to cardiovert or reduce the rate may precipitate cardiovascular collapse.* Radiofrequency ablation may be successful in experienced centres.
  - Sudden death is particularly common in this patient group, especially those with previous atrial flutter or poor hemodynamic status.
- Systemic (tricuspid) AV valve regurgitation.
  - Almost obligate. Usually progressive. TV replacement (repair rarely successful) should be considered before RV deteriorates.
  - ACE inhibitors widely used, but randomized studies are lacking.
- Systemic (R) ventricular failure
  - Common and progressive.
  - Associated with longstanding TV regurgitation, poor ventricular filling due to atrial surgery, myocardial perfusion abnormalities.
  - Management—standard heart failure therapy, but:
    —heart rate control. Tachycardia prevents ventricular filling through the restrictive surgically modified atria.
    —ACEI may not be beneficial and may impair ventricular filling.
    —conversion to arterial switch. Rarely possible beyond adolescence. See larger texts for more detail.
- Systemic or pulmonary venous pathway obstruction. Few clinical signs.
  - Systemic venous pathway obstruction may be relieved by transcatheter balloon dilatation or stenting.
  - Pulmonary venous pathway obstruction usually requires surgery.
- Baffle leak—up to 25% of the patients. Causes shunting L-to-R or R-to-L (cyanosis—increasing during exercise).
  - If clinically indicated, transcatheter closure usually successful.
- PHT—may develop in patients with late repair and/or associated VSD.

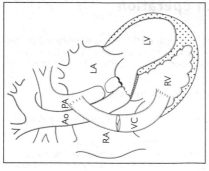

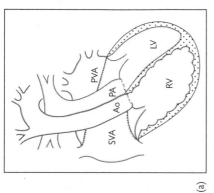

Fig. 12.2 (□ See also Plate 6) Surgical approaches to complete TGA. (a) Schematic representation of interatrial repair (Senning or Mustard operation). (b) Schematic representation of Rastelli operation. Ao aorta; LA left atrium; LV left ventricle; PA pulmonary artery; RA right atrium; RV right ventricle; VC valved conduit. Ao aorta; LV left ventricle; PA pulmonary artery; PVA pulmonary venous atrium; SVA systemic venous atrium.

Arterial switch operation

📖 See Fig. 12.3.

Now operation of choice in complete TGA. Blood is redirected at arterial level by switching the aorta and PAs, and reimplanting the coronary arteries into the neo-aortic root. Allows the MV and the LV to support the systemic circulation.

Complications of the arterial switch operation

- PA stenosis:
  - Common, due to stretching of the PAs to reach the neo-pulmonary trunk at the time of surgery.
  - Many require balloon dilation, stenting, or reoperation.
- Coronary arteries abnormalities—rare in adulthood, but obstruction of the reimplanted coronary arteries may lead to myocardial infarction and sudden death.
- Neo-aortic regurgitation—associated with aortic root dilatation. Occasionally requires reoperation.

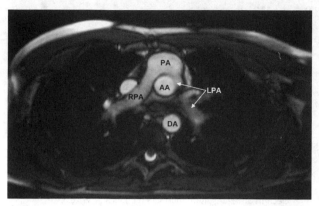

Fig. 12.3 TGA post arterial switch operation with le Compte manoeuvre. Transaxial MRI scan on a 19-year-old 4 who underwent an arterial switch operation with le Compte manoeuvre as a neonate. The le Compte manoeuvre involves bringing the PAs forward so that they lie anterior to, and straddle, the aorta. The LPA lies out of plane in this image. AA ascending aorta; DA descending aorta; PA, LPA, and RPA (L, R) pulmonary artery.

Rastelli operation

📖 See Fig. 12.2(b), p.149.

Used if TGA, large sub aortic VSD, and PS. VSD is closed so that the LV empties into the aorta. PA ligated. Conduit is placed between RV and PA. LV therefore supports the systemic circulation.

Inevitable need for redo conduit replacements and late risk of atrial and ventricular arrhythmias and complete heart block.

Follow-up of patients with TGA

- Most patients need annual follow-up.
- Clinical examination:
  - Raised JVP—PHT, baffle obstruction.
  - Mustard/Senning—parasternal heave due to systemic RV, loud palpable single S2 due to anteriorly lying aorta
  - Congestive heart failure.
  - Ejection or regurgitation murmurs (conduits or valves).
- ECG:
  - Senning/Mustard—may have junctional rhythm. RAD and RVH due to systemic RV.
  - Rastelli—RVH indicates conduit obstruction.
  - Arterial switch—should be normal.
- Echocardiography:
  - Mustard/Senning—patency of the systemic and pulmonary venous pathways, baffle leaks, degree of systemic AV valve regurgitation, systemic R ventricular function (tissue Doppler).
  - Rastelli—residual VSDs, degree of conduit stenosis, LV function.
  - Arterial switch—pulmonary arterial stenoses, degree of AR, LV function. Dobutamine stress echo if concern about coronary perfusion.
- MRI—Echo rarely provides complete information in these patients; MRI is usually needed:
  - Mustard/Senning—patency of pathways, RV function, TR severity.
  - Rastelli—conduit stenosis.
  - Arterial switch—pulmonary arterial stenoses, myocardial perfusion.
- Exercise testing:
  - Useful every 3–5 years to track changes in physical performance.
  - Mustard/Senning—chronotropic response to exercise (need for pacemaker), cyanosis (baffle leak or PHT).
  - Arterial switch—exercise-induced ischemia.
- 24-hour Holter monitoring—Senning/Mustard: tachy- and bradyarrhythmias.
- TOE—Mustard/Senning: useful if baffle stenosis or leaks are suspected; required during catheter intervention.

Exercise and sport

All TGA patients should be encouraged to exercise regularly. Mustard/Senning—avoid competitive sport and more than moderate isometric exercise. Uncomplicated arterial switch and Rastelli—no restriction.

Congenitally corrected TGA (ccTGA)

ccTGA—AV and VA discordance

Introduction
📖 See Chapters 12A, p.144 for description of connections and physiology and Fig. 12.1(b), p.145.
- Rare, <1% of all congenital heart disease.
- 95% have associated anomalies:
  - VSD with PS.
  - Ebstein (📖 see Fig.12.5).
  - AS.
  - AVSD
  - Abnormalities of situs.
  - Coarctation.
- 5% have congenital complete heart block that may also develop later in life.

Natural (unoperated) and operated history
Presentation depends on associated lesions. Isolated ccTGA may remain undiagnosed into old age. Most symptomatic by 4th decade because of failure of the systemic RV, TR, onset of complete heart block, atrial arrhythmias. Those with VSD and PS may be cyanosed.

Complications of ccTGA
Systemic TV regurgitation and systemic RV failure
TR and RV dysfunction usually co-exist. Increasing frequency in older patients. Associated with heart block, other cardiac lesions and previous heart operations.
- ACE-inhibitors may be useful, but no trial data.
- Anatomical repair (double switch or Senning–Rastelli) to restore LV to systemic circulation. Rarely possible in adults, see larger texts.
- TV replacement with a mechanical valve if RVEF ≥40%.
- Cardiac transplantation is the only option if severe TR and poor RV function and unsuitable for double-switch operation. However pulmonary vascular resistance may be too high.

Arrhythmia
- AV block may be precipitated by surgical repair, more common with increasing age.
- Sudden death rare and probably related to poor ventricular function.

Patient assessment and follow-up
Most patients need annual follow-up.

Medical history
Physical capacity, dyspnoea, palpitation, and syncope.

Clinical examination
- Parasternal heave due to the anterior systemic RV.
- Loud, palpable single S2 due to anteriorly lying aorta.
- Signs of congestive heart failure.
- TR murmur.

ECG (▢ see Fig.12.4)
- Varying degrees of AV block or evidence of pre-excitation due to accessory pathways.
- There may be L-axis deviation.
- The R and L bundles are inverted, resulting in Q waves in V1–2 and an absent Q in V5–6 (not to be misinterpreted as a previous anterior myocardial infarction).

Echocardiography
Challenging, due to frequent cardiac malposition and discordant AV, VA connections.
- A segmental approach strongly recommended (▢ see Chapter 1, p.6).
- Assessment of systemic RV function by tissue-Doppler technique.
- Quantitative echo-Doppler assessment of systemic (tricuspid) AV valve regurgitation difficult; comparison with previous studies may be useful.
- Look for Ebstein-like displacement of the mural leaflet of the TV.
- Obstruction to the subpulmonary, LV outflow tract may be multi-leveled and PA and branches may be difficult to visualize.
- Assess associated or residual cardiac lesions.

MRI
- Complementary to echo.
- More robust method to quantify systemic RV and TV function.

Exercise testing
- Useful every 3–5 years to track changes in physical performance.
- Evaluate efficacy of medical and/or surgical interventions.

24-hour Holter monitoring
Progression of heart block (need for pacemaker).

Exercise and sport
Regular, non-competitive exercise of low-to-moderate dynamic and low static intensity should be encouraged.

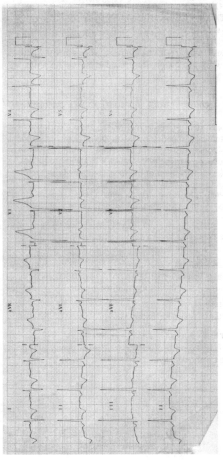

Fig 12.4 ECG of a 30-year-old with ccTGA. There is SR, RVH, and widespread T wave inversion.

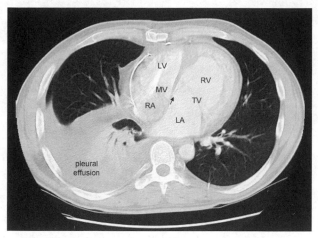

Fig. 12.5 Multislice CT scan of a 28-year-old ♂ with ccTGA. The systemic RV is dilated and hypertrophied. The interventricular septum is pushed towards the LV. There is apical displacement of the TV (arrow). The artefact across the MV is due to a pacing lead in the subpulmonary LV. There is a large R pleural effusion. LA left atrium; LV left ventricle; MV mitral valve; RA right atrium; RV right ventricle; TV tricuspid valve.

Tetralogy of Fallot and pulmonary atresia with VSD

Tetralogy of Fallot

Definition (Fig. 13.1)
The 1° abnormality is anterocephalad deviation of the outlet ventricular septum which results in the 4 abnormalities described by Fallot:
- VSD.
- Subpulmonary stenosis.
- Aorta overrides crest of interventricular septum.
- 2° RVH.

There is great morphological variation, ranging from minimal pulmonary stenosis to pulmonary atresia, and from minimal aortic override to double outlet right ventricle (DORV).

Incidence
Commonest cyanotic lesion 1:3600 livebirths; ♂ = ♀.

Associations
Cardiac associations
- 16% R aortic arch (📖 see Fig. 13.2). Particularly associated with 22q11 deletions.
- 15% persistent LSVC draining to CS:
  - Compared with 0.3% in general population, 3–10% in other patients with congenital heart disease.
  - Beware pacing—all patients with CHD should have a L arm venogram to assess systemic venous drainage before starting the procedure, to avoid the difficulty of pacing via an anomalous vein.
- Secundum ASD.
- Additional VSD.
- Aortopulmonary collaterals.

Chromosome 22 deletion
Deletion or microdeletion of chromosome 22q11 associated with broad spectrum of phenotypic abnormalities including the velocardiofacial syndrome (includes DiGeorge syndrome). Higher risk of recurrence of congenital heart disease in offspring if a 22q11 abnormality is present.

Abnormalities associated with chromosome 22q11 deletions:
- Cardiac defects:
  - Fallot with R aortic arch.
  - Truncus arteriosus.
  - Pulmonary atresia VSD.
  - Interrupted aortic arch.
- Facial—cleft palate harelip.
- Learning difficulties and psychiatric disorder

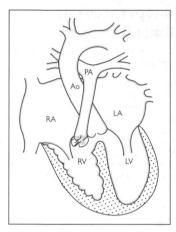

Fig 13.1 (📖 See also Plate 7) Schematic representation of unoperated tetralogy of Fallot. * deviation of outlet septum, Ao aorta; LA left atrium; LV left ventricle; PA pulmonary artery; RA right atrium; RV right ventricle.

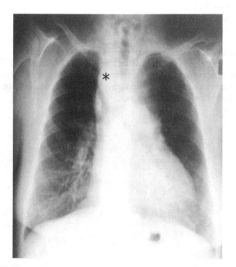

Fig. 13.2 Tetralogy of Fallot with R-sided aortic arch. Chest radiograph of a 24-year-old ♀ with repaired tetralogy of Fallot and a R-sided aortic arch (*). This anomaly is present in ~16% of patients with tetralogy of Fallot and is associated with chromosome 22q11 microdeletions.

Natural (unoperated) or shunt-palliated history

Unoperated, ~2% survive 40 years. Survival facilitated if only mild RVOTO in early life (may progress over time).

Complications—unoperated

- Complications of cyanosis (📖 see Chapter 6, pp.60–62).
- Atrial and ventricular arrhythmia.
- Progressive ascending aortic dilatation (but not the high risk of dissection associated with Marfan syndrome).
- AR—causes volume overload of both ventricles and contributes to onset of biventricular failure.
- Systemic hypertension adds additional pressure overload to both ventricles and contributes to the onset of biventricular failure.
- Endocarditis.

Physical signs—unoperated

- Cyanosis, clubbing.
- RV heave.
- Palpable thrill and loud ejection systolic murmur from RVOTO.
- Soft P2.

Investigations

Points to look for:
- ECG—RAD, RVH.
- CXR—'coeur en sabot', ↓ pulmonary vascularity, may be R aortic arch
- Echo—intracardiac anatomy and function readily identified with TTE.
- Additional information not gained from echo—PA anatomy and PA pressure and vascular resistance, presence of collaterals. MRI may replace angiography, but does not provide PA pressure data. Angiographic assessment should be made in the specialist centre prior to consideration for radical repair.

Operated history—follow up after radical repair

 See Fig. 13.3.

Radical repair involves:
- Patch closure of VSD.
- Resection of infundibular stenosis.
- Transannular patch to enlarge pulmonary valve annulus in majority of patients.

Great majority of adults with tetralogy of Fallot have undergone radical repair. Good long-term prognosis: ≥86% survival to 32 years. Morbidity likely to be better if repaired in childhood via a transatrial approach, than if repaired in adulthood or by the older transventricular approach. All at risk of late complications, therefore lifelong specialist follow up required

Complications and sequelae of radical repair
- RBBB in >99% post radical repair. The R bundle runs in the floor of the VSD and is damaged during surgical repair.
- PR—inevitable if repair included transannular patch.
- Late complete heart block may develop.
- Residual RVOTO.
- AR.
- Endocarditis.
- Arrhythmia (atrial and ventricular).
  - Atrial arrhythmia: ~30% under long-term follow up. Often scar-related intra-atrial reentry tachycardia (atrial flutter). Rapidly conducted flutter poorly tolerated and requires urgent cardioversion.
  - Ventricular arrhythmia—in up to 45% under long-term follow up.
- Sudden death, likely to be arrhythmogenic

Follow up of the patient with severe PR
Significant PR virtually universal if radical repair involved transannular patch across the RVOT. Patients usually asymptomatic for many years, but eventually RV dilation and dysfunction cause symptoms:
- Exercise intolerance.
- Atrial and ventricular arrhythmia.
- RV failure.

Signs
- Loss of sinus rhythm indicates decompensation—intervention needed.
- Elevated jugular venous pressure (JVP), hepatomegaly, and peripheral oedema—late signs indicating RV decompensation and the need for PV replacement.
- RV heave from volume-loaded RV.
- P2 soft.
- PR may be soft or inaudible (the severe regurgitant jet may be laminar and therefore inaudible).

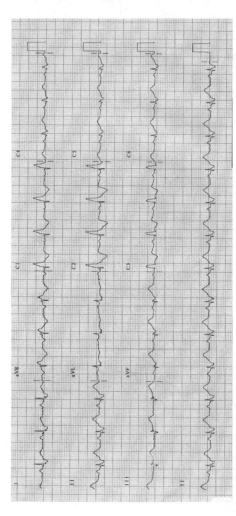

Fig. 13.3 Tetralogy of Fallot. ECG of a 22-year-old who underwent radical repair of tetralogy of Fallot aged 4. The R bundle runs in the floor of the Fallot-type VSD and is almost universally damaged at the time of surgical repair, resulting in RBBB.

Investigation
- ECG:
  - QRS duration: >180ms may indicate significantly dilated RV.
  - Atrioventricular node dysfunction: heart block.
- CXR:
  - Increasing heart size.
  - Aneurysmal RVOT or PAs.
- Echo:
  - LV, RV size and function.
  - Paradoxical IVS motion.
  - Residual VSD.
  - AR.
  - Aortic root dilation (does not carry the high risk of dissection seen in Marfan syndrome).
  - RVOTO—at subvalvar, valvar, or supravalvar level.
  - Dilated CS suggesting drainage of a persistent LSVC.
- CPEX:
  - New or more marked cardiac limitation to exercise.
  - Restrictive lung defect from associated kyphoscoliosis or previous thoracotomy: may add to symptoms and increase operative risk.
- MRI:
  - Quantification of LV and RV volume and ejection fraction.
  - Quantification of pulmonary regurgitant fraction.
  - Pulmonary arterial stenoses.
- Cardiac catheter—usually only required to relieve pulmonary arterial stenoses (balloon dilation ± stent prior to surgical valve replacement).

Timing of pulmonary valve replacement
Should probably be at 1st sign of symptoms (exercise intolerance or arrhythmia), ↑ RV volume or ↓ RV function.

Transcatheter pulmonary valve replacement now possible for patients with pre-existing valved RV–PA conduits ≤22mm diameter. Not suitable for repaired Fallots with native RVOT. No long-term follow up data yet.

Pulmonary atresia with VSD

Introduction
- Complex and heterogeneous cyanotic condition.
- Intracardiac anatomy same as Fallot, but RV outflow tract is blind ended (atretic).
- Pulmonary blood supply derived entirely from 3 types of systemic vessels:
  - Large muscular duct that resembles a collateral.
  - Diffuse plexus of small 'bronchial' arteries arising from mediastinal and intercostal arteries.
  - Large tortuous systemic arterial collaterals—MAPCAs. Arise directly from DA, its major branches, or from bronchial arteries. May connect with central PAs or supply whole segments or lobes of lung independently.

Prognosis and management depend on the pulmonary vasculature, in which there is considerable anatomical variation. Pulmonary vascular resistance depends on how many segments of lung are supplied and on the arborization pattern of the pulmonary vessels.
- If confluent PAs and MAPCAs with good arborization to all lung segments, radical repair (pink patient) possible—recruit all MAPCAs to native PAs, place RV–PA conduit, close VSD.
- If no native PAs or unfavourable pattern of MAPCAs—no or palliative surgery possible, remains cyanosed. Poor long-term outlook.

Physical signs
Similar to unoperated Fallot, plus:
- Continuous collateral murmurs.
- May have collapsing pulse.
- AR may be present.

Investigation
- CXR—R aortic arch in 25%. Typical appearance (📖 see Fig. 13.4).
- Echo—as Fallot. Colour flow Doppler indicates collateral vessels.
- Conventional angiography in specialist centre required to precisely delineate origin, degree of ostial stenosis, and intrapulmonary course of MAPCAs.
- Multislice CT and MRI useful to show relation of MAPCAs to other intrathoracic structures when planning surgery.

Late complications—unoperated or palliated
As unoperated Fallot, plus include increasing cyanosis due to:
- Development of pulmonary vascular disease in lung segments perfused at systemic pressure through non-stenosed MAPCAs.
- Stenosis of MAPCAs—may be improved by stenting.

Late complications after radical repair
As repaired Fallot, plus:
- Repeated conduit replacements
- RV failure if high pulmonary vascular resistance.

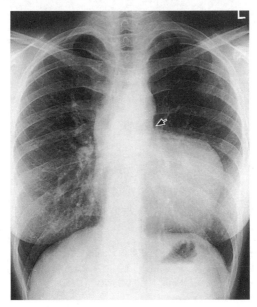

Fig 13.4 Chest radiograph of a 21-year-old woman with tetralogy of Fallot and pulmonary atresia, no central pulmonary arteries, and multiple aortopulmonary collaterals which create an abnormal pulmonary vascular pattern. The typical 'coeur on sabot' silhouette is due to right ventricular hypertrophy and the pulmonary bay where the pulmonary artery should be (arrow). Reproduced from Warrell, D et al., (2005). *Oxford Textbook of Medicine* 4th edn, with permission from Oxford University Press.

Functionally univentricular hearts and Fontan circulation

The functionally univentricular heart

Introduction
Rare and highly complex form of cyanotic congenital heart disease. The term describes a variety of cardiac malformations in which:
- There is functionally a single ventricular cavity.
- Biventricular repair is not anatomically or surgically achievable.

The ventricle may be of R or L ventricular morphology and in the majority of cases there is a 2nd rudimentary nonfunctional ventricle. Associated abnormalities are usually present:
- Abnormal atrio-ventricular and ventriculo-arterial connections.
- Atrial isomerism.
- Dextrocardia.
- Outflow tract abnormalities.

Common types of functionally univentricular heart
- Tricuspid atresia (rudimentary RV with dominant LV) (Fig. 14.1).
- Double inlet LV (Fig. 14.2)—usually with transposed great vessels ± PS.
- Unbalanced atrioventricular septal defect—often associated with atrial isomerism.
- Pulmonary atresia with intact septum and hypoplastic RV.
- Hypoplastic left heart syndrome (□ see Hypoplastic left heart syndrome (HLHS), p.188).

Presentation
- In neonatal life with cyanosis.
- Presentation depends on the pulmonary blood flow:
  - Too little pulmonary blood flow leads to profound hypoxaemia and circulatory collapse, requiring emergency palliation.
  - Too much pulmonary blood flow leads to pulmonary vascular remodeling and PHT if left untreated.
- Initial management is to regulate the pulmonary blood flow:
  - If pulmonary blood flow is too high, flow is restricted by banding the PA or
  - If pulmonary blood flow is too little, flow is augmented with a systemic-pulmonary shunt.
  - Rarely, the circulation is well balanced and no early intervention is needed.

Left untreated the natural history of univentricular hearts is very poor and few survive early childhood.

Management
- Physiological and anatomical considerations:
- Correction to a biventricular circulation is not feasible.
- All therapeutic strategies are palliative.
- Requires low pulmonary vascular resistance for good outcome.
- SVC flow accounts for 70% of venous return in infant.
- Aim to improve cyanosis, effort tolerance, and survival.

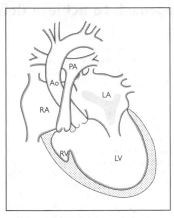

Fig.14.1 (📖 See also Plate 8) Schematic representation of tricuspid atresia. Systemic venous blood leaves the RA via an atrial septal defect and mixes with pulmonary venous blood in the LA. The LV thus supports both the systemic and pulmonary circulations and the patient is cyanosed. The rudimentary RV does not play a functional role. Ao aorta; LA left atrium; LV left ventricle; PA pulmonary artery; RA right atrium; RV right ventricle.

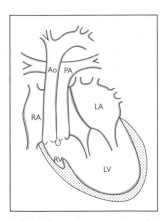

Fig. 14.2 (📖 See also Plate 9) Schematic representation of double inlet LV with VA discordance. Both atria connect to the LV via the tricuspid and mitral valves, so that systemic and pulmonary venous blood mix in the LV and the patient is cyanosed. The LV supports both the systemic and pulmonary circulations. The aorta arises from the rudimentary RV via the VSD. If the VSD is restrictive, it creates obstruction to systemic blood flow. Ao aorta; LA left atrium; LV left ventricle; PA pulmonary artery; RA right atrium; RV right ventricle; VA ventriculoarterial; VSD ventricular septal defect.

Staged approach to achieve definitive palliation

- The end result of this approach is a Fontan-type circulation (Fig. 14.3).
- There are many variations of the Fontan operation.
- Current practice is a staged approach. Number of stages depends on initial anatomy. Older patients may have had single-stage approach.

Initial stage

- Control of pulmonary blood flow:
  - PA band to limit flow.
  - Systemic arterial shunt to increase flow.
- Secure unobstructed systemic outflow (e.g. in AS). The Damus–Kaye–Stanzel procedure involves creating a direct connection between the AA and the mPA. The mPA is divided before the bifurcation and anastomosed into an opening made into the facing side of the AA—thus, flow from the functionally single ventricle reaches the aorta via both the aortic and pulmonary valves. Pulmonary blood flow is via a shunt from the aorta or a conduit from the ventricle. The technique is used to overcome complex types of aortic and sub-aortic obstruction that cannot be relieved from within the heart.

Cavopulmonary shunt (Glenn operation)

- Systemic venous shunt (SVC is disconnected from the heart and connected directly to the PAs—a cavopulmonary anastomosis).
- Only possible when the PVR is low (typically after 3–4 months of age).
- Classical Glenn—RPA disconnected from main PA, SVC disconnected from RA. SVC to RPA connected end-to-end. Historical, no longer performed.
- Bidirectional Glenn—SVC disconnected from RA. SVC connected to RPA end-to-side anastomosis. RPA left in continuity with main PA.

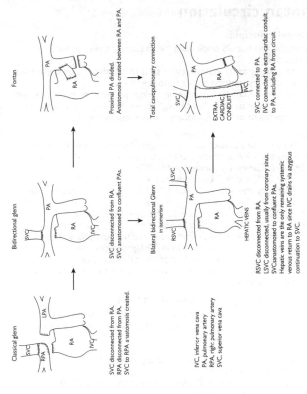

Classical glenn

SVC disconnected from RA.
RPA disconnected from PA.
SVC to RPA anastomosis created.

IVC, inferior vena cava
PA, pulmonary artery
RPA, right pulmonary artery
SVC, superior vena cava

Bidirectional glenn

SVC disconnected from RA.
SVC anastomosed to confluent PAs.

Bilateral bidirectional Glenn in isomerism

RSVC disconnected from RA.
LSVC disconnected, usually from coronary sinus.
SVC anastomosed to confluent PAs.
Hepatic veins are the only remaining systemic venous return to RA since IVC drains via azygous continuation to SVC.

Fontan

Proximal PA divided.
Anastomosis created between RA and PA.

Total cavopulmonary connection

SVC connected to PA.
IVC connected via extra-cardiac conduit to PA, excluding RA from circuit.

Fig. 14.3 Evolution of Fontan and total cavopulmonary connection.

Fontan circulation

General principles

- Uses the functionally single ventricle to support the systemic circulation
- Directs the systemic venous return straight into the PAs i.e. there is no subpulmonary ventricle so flow into the PAs is:
  - Passive—relies on high systemic venous pressures to provide a head of pressure to drive flow through the pulmonary vasculature.
  - Dependent on low pulmonary vascular resistance.

There are 2 different surgical approaches:

- Atriopulmonary connection—the original Fontan procedure, many variations e.g. RA appendage connected directly to the PA.
- Total cavopulmonary connection (TCPC):
  - Both SVC and IVC are connected separately to the PAs using a Glenn for the SVC and routing the IVC with either a lateral tunnel within the RA or with an extra-cardiac conduit.
  - TCPC has been the procedure of choice since ~1990.
  - The TCPC is frequently fenestrated (i.e. small communication created between the Fontan circuit and the pulmonary venous atrium) to act as an escape valve for high systemic venous pressures. Result is a (small) R–L shunt that causes a degree of desaturation but benefit is to offset high venous pressures and improve systemic cardiac output.

Post Fontan surgery (📖 see Figs. 14.4–6)

The physiological consequence of a Fontan-type operation is a circulation with high systemic venous pressures and passive pulmonary blood flow. This leads to:

- RA dilatation.
- Poor flow from atrium to PA with energy dissipation.
- Loss of effort tolerance.
- Atrial arrhythmias common often with life-threatening consequences.

TCPC may mitigate against some of these complications, by bypassing the RA. However, all types of Fontan surgery rely on passive flow into PAs and produce a chronic low cardiac output state.

Physical examination

- Cyanosis and clubbing may be present if fenestration or collateral vessels.
- Pulse should be regular (check ECG) but radial pulse may be absent if previous shunt.
- JVP usually is elevated ≥2cm due to high Fontan pressures (typically CVP is ~15mmHg compared with normal mRA pressure ~ 5 mmHg.
- Auscultation will not reveal murmur of underlying congenital cardiac malformation but PSM may indicate atrioventricular valve regurgitation (AVVR). Often single 2nd sound.

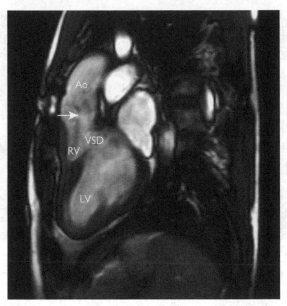

Fig. 14.4 Double inlet LV with VA discordance, post Fontan operation. MRI scan of a 24-year-old 4 with double inlet LV and ventriculo-arterial discordance. This sagittal section shows the anterior aorta arising from a rudimentary anterior RV. Blood passes from the LV through a large VSD. There is mild AR (arrow). The patient has undergone a Fontan procedure (not shown on this image). Ao aorta; LV left ventricle; RV right ventricle; VSD ventricular septal defect.

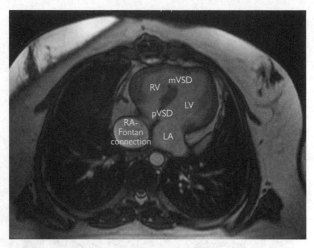

Fig. 14.5 TGA post Fontan operation. MRI scan (transaxial view) of a 22-year-old with TGA, PS, straddling MV and inlet perimembanous and muscular VSDs. The straddling MV (straddle not seen in this view) rendered biventricular repair impossible, so she underwent palliation with an atriopulmonary Fontan operation aged 6 years. LA left atrium; LV left ventricle; mVSD muscular ventricular septal defect; pVSD perimembranous ventricular septal defect; RA right atrium; RV right ventricle.

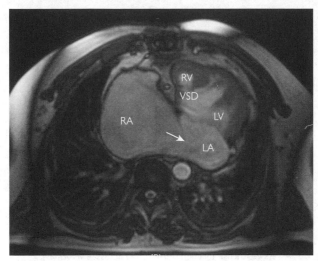

Fig. 14.6 Tricuspid atresia post Fontan operation. Transaxial section MRI scan of a 41-year-old with tricuspid atresia who underwent a bidirectional Glenn operation aged 10, and an atriopulmonary Fontan operation aged 21 years. There is a single atrioventricular (mitral) valve that connects to the LV. The rudimentary RV lies anteriorly. The atrial septum bows to the L (arrow) as a result of elevated pressures in the hugely dilated RA. LA left atrium; LV left ventricle; VSD ventricular septal defect; RA right atrium; RV right ventricle.

- May have parasternal heave if single RV.
- Normal to feel liver edge.
- Ascites or pulmonary effusion should be investigated as may be a sign of protein-losing enteropathy (PLE)
- Chest should be clear but restrictive lung defects are common owing to previous thorocotomies.

Investigation
- ECG
  - Check in SR. Give patient copy of ECG to carry with them.
  - May have axis deviation dependent on ventricular morphology.
  - May show atrial hypertrophy if atriopulmonary Fontan.
  - Intra-atrial reentry tachycardia may be mistaken for SR and requires prompt cardioversion (📖 see Chapter 16. p.204).
- CXR:
  - May indicate previous surgical procedures (thoracotomy).
  - To look for kyphoscoliosis—perform lung function tests if present.
  - Give indication of situs and isomerism—gas bubble, symmetry of bronchi.
- Echocardiography—routine TTE:
  - Confirm congenital abnormality, situs and ventricular morphology best subcostal, A4C and PLAX views.
  - Assess ventricular function (MAPSE/TAPSE/tissue velocities).
  - Assess degree of AVVR.
  - Ventricular outflow tract obstruction.
  - Aortic incompetence.
  - Turbulent pulmonary venous return.
- Echocardiography—TOE:
  - Not routine, often requires GA.
  - For investigation of failing Fontan.
  - Evaluate AVVR and Fontan pathway.
  - Exclude pulmonary venous obstruction.
- Cardiac MRI:
  - Good to:
    —assess flow in Fontan pathway.
    —assess ventricular function and anatomy.
    —exclude pulmonary venous obstruction.
  - No pressure data.
  - Claustrophobia is a problem.
- Metabolic exercise testing (📖 see Chapter 3, p.38)
  - Useful in defining cause of exercise limitation e.g. pulmonary or cardiac.
  - Good Fontan generally has ~70% predicted MVO_2.
  - Not been evaluated in terms of prognosis in congenital heart disease.
- Blood tests:
  - Routine FBC—Hb may be raised and platelets ↓ reflecting cyanosis.
  - Routine U&Es and LFTs—impaired renal function is cause for concern, LFTs often mildly deranged due to hepatic congestion.
  - If albumin/total protein is low, then investigate for PLE.

Complications following Fontan surgery

The main complications of this circulation are:
- Atrial arrhythmias.
- SA node dysfunction.
- Systemic AV valve regurgitation.
- Ventricular dysfunction.
- Fontan pathway obstruction.
- Pulmonary venous pathway obstruction.
- Cyanosis (due to opening up of venous collaterals from the Fontan circuit to the pulmonary veins and/or flow through the fenestration).
- Development of subaortic stenosis.
- Thromboembolism.
- Hepatic dysfunction.
- PLE due to high mesenteric venous pressures.

Management of the post-Fontan patient (📖 see Fig. 14.7)

General management points

- All adult patients should be anticoagulated with warfarin.
  - The flow in the Fontan circuit is passive not pulsatile and therefore spontaneous thrombus formation is possible.
  - Protein C and S deficiency is common increasing risk of thrombosis.
  - Micro thrombi in the distal pulmonary arterioles will lead to ↑ pulmonary vascular resistance, detrimental to the Fontan circuit.
- Avoid dehydration:
  - Dehydration reduces the filling pressure in the Fontan circuit and reduce pre-load in the single ventricle, compromising cardiac output and systemic BP.
  - Rehydrate during intercurrent illness.
  - If nil by mouth (NBM), give IV fluids, 1L normal saline over 12 hours.
- GA:
  - Avoid unless absolutely necessary; requires *senior* anaesthetist who understand the Fontan circulation.
  - If NBM hydrate by IV fluids, 1L normal saline over 12 hours.
  - All anesthetic agents cause systemic vasodilatation.
  - +ve pressure ventilation reduces venous return and therefore cardiac output.
  - Lack of pre-load recruitment makes low systemic vascular resistance (SVR) difficult to overcome.
  - Have metaraminol available to maintain SVR and systemic BP during anesthesia.
- Management of atrial flutter/tachycardia (📖 see Chapter 16, p.204 for detailed management):
  - A common and life-threatening event.
  - Mechanism is a scar-related intra-atrial reentrant tachycardia (IART), or atypical atrial flutter.
  - Patient presents with palpitations.
  - Rhythm is often regular and often not rapid (HR 90–120).
  - ECG may be mistaken for SR, *compare* with ECG in normal rhythm (ensure patients carries a copy of their normal ECG at all times).
  - Do not attempt chemical cardioversion as may trigger rapid conduction and circulatory collapse.
  - *Arrange prompt cardioversion (sedation only is safe)*.
  - Long-term prevention with amiodarone is often necessary (check thyroid function every 3 months: thyrotoxicosis common late side effect, may cause permanent deterioration in functional status).
  - Electrophysiology study and RFA of multiple scar-related pathways may lead to reduction in symptoms.

A: sinus rhythm

B: interatrial re-entry tachycardia

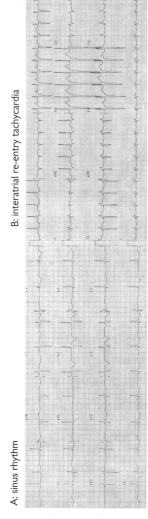

Fig. 14.7 Atrial tachyarrhythmia post Fontan operation for tricuspid atresia.

A 24-year-old 4 who underwent Fontan palliation for tricuspid atresia in childhood had episodes of interatrial tachyarrhythmia. 12-lead ECG (a) shows him in sinus rhythm. He had been advised to seek urgent medical assistance if he developed palpitation. He began to feel unwell and breathless with palpitation, but delayed for 2 days before presenting to a local emergency department. His ECG (b) showed an IART but was misdiagnosed as sinus tachycardia and no treatment was given. The following day he had a cardiac arrest and could not be resuscitated. At-risk patients should be advised to seek help rapidly if palpitation occurs, given copies of their ECG to carry, and a letter detailing their diagnosis and instructions for emergency cardioversion.

The failing Fontan

Definition

- Without Fontan-type surgery majority of single ventricle patients would not survive into adulthood.
- Fontan circuit is by its nature palliative.
- Fontan circulation is a low cardiac output state.
- Effort tolerance is limited even in 'well' patients.
- Signs of 'failure':
  - Ventricular dysfunction.
  - Reduced effort tolerance.
  - Arrhythmias.
  - PLE.

Why it happens

Ventricular dysfunction

- ↑ afterload leads to hypertrophy of ventricle.
- Limited pre-load recruitment leads to diastolic dysfunction.
- Ventricular hypertrophy leads to systolic dysfunction.
- *Management:*
  - No data to support conventional therapy e.g. ACE inhibitors, beta-blockade, spironolactone.
  - Empiric treatment with beta-blockade and spironolactone may help symptoms.
  - O_2 therapy may help.
  - Diuretics should be used with caution due to risk of hypovolaemia.
  - Exclude underlying causes e.g. outflow tract obstruction, AVVR, Fontan pathway obstruction, pulmonary venous obstruction, paroxysmal arrhythmias.

Reduced effort tolerance

- Impaired ventricular function.
- AVVR (often due to annular dilatation) leads to ↑ left atrial pressure.
- Further reduces the effective gradient down which blood flows.
- Further reduces cardiac output.
- *Management:*
  - Ensure no lung involvement.
  - Restrictive lung defect may benefit from O_2 therapy and/or non-invasive ventilation.
  - Exercise program may improve symptoms of breathlessness.

Pulmonary vascular remodelling

- Distal muscularization of pulmonary arterioles occurs:
  → ↑ pulmonary vascular resistance.
  → ↓ flow through lungs.
  → failure to pre-load recruit leads to lower cardiac output.
- *Management:*
  - Impossible to prove without lung biopsy (*not* recommended).
  - Empiric therapy with targeted pulmonary vasodilator therapy may help, but no data available.

Atrial arrhythmias
- Multiple scars related to suture lines and bypass cannulation—provide circuits for macro-rentrant tachycardias.
- ↑ incidence with age.
- Associated with decline in ventricular function.
- *Management:*
  - 📖 see Chapter 16, p.204 for acute management.
  - Often require amiodarone to suppress arrhythmia.
  - May be triggered by excessive alcohol.
  - Consider EP studies in all patients with flutter.

PLE
- Particular problem for Fontan patients.
- High mesenteric venous pressure → protein loss into gut.
- Assessed by demonstrating low serum albumin, immunoglobulins, and raised faecal alpha-1 antitrypsin levels from fresh stool sample (contact local biochemistry department for details of sampling).
  - Low albumin, total protein and immunoglobulin levels leads to effusions, ascites, and dependent oedema, malnutrition, recurrent cellulites, and septicaemia.
  - No reliably effective treatment; *may benefit from:*
    —daily unfractionated SC heparin.
    —systemic steroids.
    —targeted pulmonary vasodilator therapy.
    —fenestration of Fontan pathway.
  - 50% 5-year mortality. Seek expert help.

Long-term outcome of Fontan surgery
- Long-term outcome is not known.
- Current adult patients are the pioneers of this operation.
- Complications, as already discussed, will inevitably → significant morbidity and mortality.
- Fontan patients form a small proportion of the total number of patients with congenital heart disease but account for 50% of emergency admissions.
- Prompt management of their medical emergencies prevents premature deaths.

Hypoplastic left heart syndrome (HLHS)

- Complex form of functionally univentricular circulation characterized by varying degrees of hypoplasia of the LV and aorta, associated with aortic and mitral atresia or stenosis.
- Relies on the morphological RV to support the systemic circulation.

Stage I (Norwood) procedure

- Requires complex neonatal surgery. Aim: to use the RV and mPA to reconstruct the systemic outflow tract and then provide pulmonary blood flow with a systemic–pulmonary artery shunt.
- Without the Norwood procedure the condition is not compatible with life.

Stage II (Glenn)

A Glenn shunt is performed at ~6 months.

Stage III (Fontan) (Fig. 14.8)

- Final definitive palliation to a Fontan circulation around 5–6 years.
- Survivors have a Fontan circulation with a systemic RV and coronary circulation arising from an often diminutive aorta.
- Procedure only developed in the 1980s so population is much younger than other adult Fontan survivors. Long-term complications unknown, but likely to be those of any Fontan, plus:
  - Coarctation repair site—recoarctation?
  - LPA—stenosis?
  - ASD—restrictive?
  - Coronaries from diminutive aorta—ischaemia?
  - Systemic RV—dysfunction?
  - Systemic tricuspid valve—regurgitation?

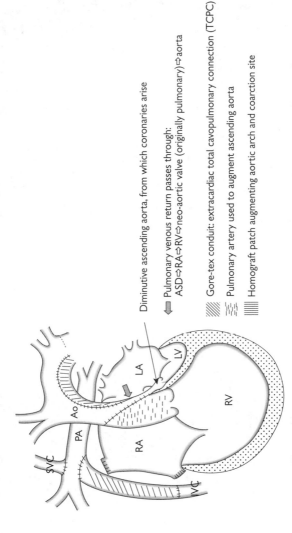

Diminutive ascending aorta, from which coronaries arise

Pulmonary venous return passes through:
ASD⇨RA⇨RV⇨neo-aortic valve (originally pulmonary)⇨aorta

Gore-tex conduit: extracardiac total cavopulmonary connection (TCPC)

Pulmonary artery used to augment ascending aorta

Homograft patch augmenting aortic arch and coarction site

Fig. 14.8 (◻ See also Plate 10) Schematic representation of hypoplastic left heart following Stage 3 Fontan palliation. Ao aorta; IVC inferior vena cava; LA left atrium; LV left ventricle; PA pulmonary artery; RA right atrium; RV right ventricle; SVC superior vena cava.

Chapter 15

Rare conditions presenting in adulthood

Coronary anomalies

📖 See Table 15.1.

Definition

- Rare.
- Occur in isolation or with associated congenital cardiac lesions.
- Clinical significance depends on potential of the anomaly to cause ischaemia and sudden death.
- Ischaemia is main indication for surgical repair and is associated with:
  - Anomalous proximal coronary course between aorta and pulmonary trunk.
  - An intramural proximal segment of the anomalous coronary artery inside the aortic wall.
  - Acute angulation between origin of anomalous coronary artery and the aortic wall.
  - Anomalous coronary artery arising from pulmonary trunk.

Left coronary artery from pulmonary artery

- Rare, usually presents in infancy with myocardial ischaemia and LV failure when pulmonary vascular resistance decreases.
- 10–15% survive to adulthood because they develop adequate intercoronary collateral circulation.
- Adult presentation:
  - Asymptomatic.
  - Myocardial ischaemia or MR due to papillary muscle dysfunction.
- Surgical repair indicated.

Congenital coronary arteriovenous fistulae

- Fistulous coronary artery branch communicates directly with RV in 40%, RA in 25%, PA 15%, rarely SVC or PV.
- Survival to adulthood usual, but longevity reduced if large fistula, coronary steal phenomenon, and myocardial ischaemia
- Symptoms ↑ with age. Risk of endocarditis, heart failure, arrhythmia, myocardial ischaemia and infarction, and sudden death.
- Surgical repair recommended unless trivial isolated shunt. Some smaller fistulae amenable to transcatheter device occlusion.

Investigation

- Congenital anomalies should be considered in adults <50 years with symptoms of ischaemia, LV or papillary muscle dysfunction.
- Assess ischaemia—exercise test, echo (± stress), 24-hour ECG tape.
- Assess anatomy—selective angiography and multislice CT may be required to delineate precise course of anomalous vessels.

Table 15.1 Major types of coronary anomaly

Anomalous origin from inappropriate aortic sinus or coronary vessel	LMS: absent (separate origins of LAD and Cx)
	LAD: from R aortic sinus or RCA
	Cx: absent, or from R aortic sinus or RCA
	RCA: from L or posterior aortic sinus, or LAD
	Single coronary artery from R or L aortic sinus
Anomalous origin from other systemic artery (rare)	Innominate, subclavian, internal mammary, carotid, bronchial arteries, or DA
Anomalous origin from PA	
Coronary arteriovenous fistulae	

Cx circumflex; DA descending aorta; LAD left anterior descending; LMS left main stem; PA pulmonary artery; RCA right coronary artery.

Sinus of valsalva aneurysm

📖 See Fig. 15.1.

Definition and natural history

- Dilatation or enlargement of ≥1 of the aortic sinuses.
- Unruptured aneurysm rarely symptomatic, but may cause obstruction—chest pain, palpitation.
- Aneurysm may progress and rupture:
  - Non-coronary sinus usually into RA.
  - R coronary sinus into RA or RV.
- Rupture usually in early adulthood, sometimes with endocarditis:
  - Sudden rupture—tearing chest pain, dyspnoea, heart and renal failure, loud *continuous* murmur.
  - Small perforations may be asymptomatic.

Management

Unruptured

- Monitor with yearly echo if asymptomatic.
- If causing symptoms, surgical repair.

Ruptured

- Diagnosis clinical—typical history and murmur.
- Confirm site with echo and angiography.
- Surgical or transcatheter repair required.

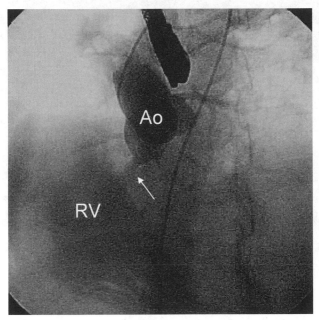

Fig. 15.1 Ruptured Sinus of Valsalva aneurysm. Aortogram of 36-year-old ♀ with ruptured sinus of Valsalva aneurysm. There is a jet of contrast from the ruptured sinus into the RV. An echo probe is positioned in the oesophagus. The ruptured aneurysm was closed using a duct occluder device. Ao aorta, RV, right ventricle.

Part 3

General management issues of adult congenital heart disease

Emergencies

Introduction

There are a number of ACHD emergencies in which quick and simple management can prevent unnecessary morbidity or mortality. Senior in-house help must always be requested and advice sought from a specialist ACHD unit.

Haemoptysis in a cyanotic patient

📖 see also Chapter 6, pp.58–62.

This is one of the leading causes of death, especially in the presence of PHT, and must be managed appropriately immediately:
- A, B, C.
- Resuscitate the patient.
- IV access with air-filter (to prevent paradoxical embolism due to R-to-L shunt).
- Bloods for FBC, clotting, X-match (**must inform haematology**).
- Keep patient NBM.
- Lower BP:
  - Remember that brachial artery BP = PA pressure in Eisenmenger syndrome.
  - Important to lower pressure in bleeding pulmonary vessel.
  - Give IV β blocker.
  - Do not give vasodilating antihypertensives that will increase the |R-to-L shunt and exacerbate hypoxia.
  - Use benzodiazepines ± opiates to keep patient calm.
- If severe haemoptysis, consider selective intubation.
- If massive haemoptysis, ensure adequate opiates so patient is not distressed.
- Liaise with specialist ACHD centre—patient may need urgent transfer.
- Urgent CT scan—involve congenital interventional cardiologist; there may be a vessel to embolize or coil.
- Establish patient diagnosis/recent intervention/surgery.

Possible causes of haemoptysis

Depends on anatomy. Consider:
- Embolism of *in situ* PA thrombus—pulmonary embolism from other sources such as DVT is unlikely.
- Bleeding from pulmonary arteriovenous malformations.
- Bleeding collateral vessels.
- Chest infection.

Other emergencies and pitfalls to avoid in cyanotic heart disease

📖 see Chapter 6, pp.56–62.

- Avoid
  - Iatrogenic renal failure.
  - Paradoxical embolism.
  - Increasing cyanosis with vasodilators.
- Maintain appropriately high haemoglobin for optimum O_2-carrying capacity.
- Avoid dehydration—give IV fluids through air filter when NBM.
- Management of tachyarrhymias.
- Management of cerebral abscess.

Haemoptysis or haematemesis in patient with repaired coarctation

📖 see also Chapter 10, pp.118–121.

Beware

Assume represents erosion of aortic aneurysm to form an aorto-bronchial or aorto-oesophageal fistula—patients with post Dacron patch repair of coarctation most at risk; aneurysm develops at suture lines.

Management

- A, B, C.
- Resuscitate the patient.
- IV access.
- Bloods for FBC, clotting, X-match.
- Keep patient NBM, monitored.
- *Urgent* contrast CT or MRI scan.
- *Avoid* invasive tests (bronchoscopy, upper GI endoscopy, aortography) because of risk of causing catastrophic haemorrhage.
- *Liaise with specialist ACHD centre*—patient needs urgent transfer for emergency surgery or aortic stenting.

Tachyarrhythmias

📖 See Fig. 16.1.

Patients with surgical correction result in surgical scars which can act as a focus for arrhythmias. Certain patient groups, particularly Fontan and Mustard/Senning patients or those with impaired function do not tolerate tachyarrhythmias for long. There is a high risk of death in these patients with arrhythmias and these patients require **urgent** DC cardioversion, **not** pharmacological therapy which is potentially lethal.

Common precipitating factors for atrial arrhythmias include alcohol, drug abuse, fatigue, emotion, unaccustomed overexertion, thyrotoxicosis (beware amiodarone).

Why atrial tachyarrhythmias are so dangerous

TGA Mustard/Senning (📖 Chapter 12, p.148)
- Flutter increasingly common with age and ventricular dysfunction.
- Restrictive atrial pathways mean that ventricular filling is compromised at rapid heart rates.
- Flutter may conduct 1:1—a heart rate of 300bpm may be fatal in this group.
- Failure to give IV fluids, or giving IV antiarrhythmics may cause cardiovascular collapse from which patient cannot be resuscitated.

Fontan (📖 Chapter 14, p.171)
- IART/atypical flutter) is common, especially in atriopulmonary Fontan with dilated RA.
- The Fontan circulation relies on a very small pressure drop across the pulmonary circulation, permitting systemic venous blood to cross the pulmonary vascular bed into the LA and then into the ventricle. During flutter, the LA pressure rises and impedes blood flow into the ventricle → *cardiac output falls.*
- If mismanaged, flutter may be fatal:
  - If no IV fluids are given, the systemic venous pressure falls, further reducing forward flow across the pulmonary circulation → *cardiac output falls further.*
  - Antiarrhythmics e.g. IV β blockers and flecainide are very unlikely to cardiovert the patient, but may produce profound hypotension → *cardiac output falls.*
  - If vasodilator anaesthetic agents are not given cautiously, remembering that the circulation time in this situation is very slow, the consequent vasodilation further reduces systemic venous pressure → *cardiac output falls.*
  - +ve pressure ventilation raises intra-thoracic pressure and reduces systemic venous return still further → *cardiac output falls* → patient cannot be resuscitated.

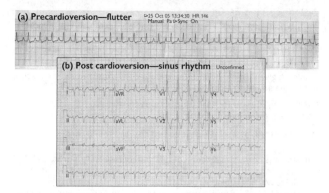

Fig. 16.1 Atrial flutter post Mustard repair of TGA. A 26-year-old ♂ who underwent Mustard repair of TGA in infancy presented hypotensive to the emergency department with syncopal palpitation of 3 hours duration. The rhythm strip (a) shows atrial flutter with 2:1 block. He reverted to sinus rhythm with urgent DC cardioversion (b) There is R axis deviation and R ventricular dominance.

Patient-carried ECGs

Patients with complex congenital heart disease often have very abnormal baseline ECGs, and interpreting them in an emergency can be difficult. Failure to recognize loss of sinus rhythm can result in the patient dying.

All patients with congenital heart disease and abnormal resting ECGs should be given a miniaturized (laminated) copy to carry on their person, so that the admitting team can compare it with the admission ECG.

Alternatively, the centre that usually cares for the patient should help in interpreting the admission ECG

Management of atrial flutter/ventricular tachycardia

- A, B, C.
- If patient is compromised, urgent DC cardioversion (ALS protocol).
- IV access and NBM.
- IV fluids with air-filter line.
- Check K^+, Mg^{2+}, TFTs, C-reactive protein (CRP), FBC, biochemistry, and international normalized ratio (INR).
- Move to CCU and monitor.
- Inform Senior/Cardiology and specialist ACHD centre.
- May need TOE if INR subtherapeutic or >24 hours duration (AF/flutter) *but* do not delay cardioversion if patient compromised.
- Liaise with anaesthetics SpR at least (preferably cardiac)—need to inform about cardiac anatomy and physiology and need for urgency.
- Avoid vasodilating anaesthetic.
- DC cardioversion (external pads) as ALS protocol.
- Need to monitor following cardioversion for at least 6 hours and investigate the reason for arrhythmia (alcohol, intercurrent infection, non-compliance, clinical deterioration, baffle obstruction etc.).
- Liaise with specialist ACHD centre re: discharge medication and consideration of ablation referral/further investigation.
- Obtain old ECGs and give patient copy of arrhythmia and discharge ECG.

Contraception and pregnancy

Introduction[1-3]

Heart disease is the largest single cause of maternal death in the UK[4]. The number and complexity of survivors of congenital heart disease well enough to consider pregnancy is growing. The maternal risk amongst this population varies from being no different to that of the general population, to carrying a high risk of long-term morbidity and >40% risk of death.

General principles

All adolescent ♀ and ♀ of child-bearing age with congenital heart disease should have access to specialist advice (NB in this context, 'specialist' = a cardiologist with expertise in both congenital heart disease and cardiac disease in pregnancy, as well as in contraception in heart disease).
Advice should include:
- For the adolescent ♀:
  - Future childbearing potential.
  - Contraceptive options.
- For all women:
  - Awareness of likely maternal risk.
  - Contraception.
- Pre-pregnancy counselling:
  - Maternal risk.
  - Fetal risk.
  - Optimize maternal condition to reduce maternal and fetal risk before pregnancy.
- Antenatal, intrapartum, and postpartum care:
  - In a joint congenital cardiac and obstetric high-risk clinic for high-risk conditions.
  - Multidisciplinary team—specialist cardiologist, obstetrician, anaesthetist, haematologist, midwife, congenital cardiac nurse specialist.

1 Thorne SA, MacGregor AE, Nelson Piercy C (2006). Risk of contraception and pregnancy in heart disease education. *Heart* **92**, 1520–5.

2 Thorne SA (2004). Pregnancy in heart disease. *Heart* **90**(4), 450–6.

3 Steer PJ, Gatzoulis MA, Baker P (eds.) (2006). *Heart Disease in Pregnancy*. RCOG Press.

4 Lewis G (ed.) (2004). *Why Mothers Die. 6th report of the Confidential Enquiries into Maternal Deaths in the UK.* Royal College Obstetrics Gynaecology: London. ⏚ www.cemach.org.uk

Contraception

For the majority of ♀, contraception is merely a method to conveniently space pregnancies. By contrast for many ♀ with congenital heat disease it is a method of preventing a potentially life-threatening condition. Advice should be offered to all ♀ of childbearing age with heart disease.

The cardiovascular safety and contraceptive efficacy of each contraceptive method must be taken into account for each congenital cardiac lesion.

In general, family planning specialists lack expertise in congenital heart disease. The cardiologist must therefore liaise with the family planning agencies and have a sound understanding of the risk and efficacy profile of the different contraceptive methods and their suitability for each cardiac lesion.

Contraceptive methods

Barrier methods

- No cardiovascular risk.
- Low efficacy—user dependent.
- Prevents sexually transmitted infection therefore encourage use in conjunction with other methods.

Oestrogen-containing preparations

- Includes combined oral contraceptive pill (COC), skin patches (vaginal ring and injectable not yet licensed in UK).
- Risk of venous and arterial thromboembolism therefore contraindicated in many conditions—📖 see Table 17.1.
- Good efficacy.

Progestogen-only methods

- Not prothrombotic, so no hormonal cardiovascular risk. However may be risk at time of insertion.
- Efficacy varies between methods.
- Menstrual effects vary between methods; all may cause initial irregular bleeding which may be unacceptable. They may be associated with subsequent (reversible) amenorrhoea: an advantage to cyanotic or anticoagulated ♀ in whom menorrhagia is common.

Table 17.1 Contraindications to COC

Risk of thromboembolism

Dilated cardiac chambers
e..g. dilated LA with MV disease, dilated cardionyopathy

Mechanical valve

Arrhythmia especially atrial fibrillation

Fontan

PHT—any cause

Previous thromboembolism

Additional risk of paradoxical embolism

Cyanotic heart disease

Unoperated ASD

Oral preparations

Standard progestogen only pill—POP, minipill
- No cardiovascular risk.
- Poor efficacy—do not use in ♀ for whom pregnancy carries significant risk.
- Irregular bleeding may resolve after initial few cycles.

Cerazette®—new desogestrel containing pill
- No cardiovascular risk.
- Efficacy at least as good as COC.
- Irregular bleeding may resolve after initial few cycles.

Long acting preparations

Depo-Provera®
- No cardiovascular risk, but delivery is by 3-monthly deep IM injection so risk of haematoma on warfarin.
- Efficacy good. However, fertility may return rapidly—failure often due to late repeat injections.
- Irregular bleeding may resolve after initial few cycles and be followed by amenorrhoea.

Implanon®
- No cardiovascular risk. Silicon rod inserted subdermally, needs replacing every 3 years.
- Efficacy better than sterilization.
- Irregular bleeding may be followed by amenorrhoea, but in a few ♀, bleeding is heavy and prolonged and requires removal of the rod.

Mirena IUS®
- Progestogen eluting intrauterine device (IUD).
- Cardiovascular risk confined to time of insertion, which should be by a skilled operator, especially for nulliparous ♀.
  - 5% risk of vagal reaction at time of insertion—it is contraindicated in PHT, Fontan circulation, and cyanotic heart disease where a vagal reaction carries a risk of cardiovascular collapse. However, if other methods not acceptable, the risk of insertion by a skilled operator may outweigh the risk of pregnancy.
  - Risk of endocarditis confined to time of insertion. Lower risk than traditional IUD. Current UK guidelines do not recommend antibiotic prophylaxis at insertion.
  - Efficacy better than sterilization.
  - Irregular bleeding often followed by amenorrhoea.
- Traditional copper IUD:
  - Cardiovascular risk as Mirena.
  - Efficacy good but less effective than Mirena
  - Painful menorrhagia common.

- Sterilization:
  - ♂ sterilization rarely appropriate:
    —assumes monogamy.
    —♂ likely to outlive ♀ partner with congenital heart disease.
  - Laparoscopic ♀ sterilization:
    —procedure carries a risk in those for whom pregnancy is the highest risk.
    —less effective than Mirena and Implanon®.
- Essure®—new hysteroscopic stent-based technique. Risks likely to be confined to time of procedure.

Preconception

Maternal risks

In order to provide counselling, an up-to-date assessment of the ♀'s condition and functional capacity is required. Information needed includes thorough history and examination, ECG, Echo, CPEX. Additional information may be needed—24-hour ECG, MRI, cardiac catheterization.

Risks are additive and likely to increase with increasing maternal age, especially for those with complex disease e.g. with systemic RV.

Canadian risk score for women with pre existing heart disease[1]

- A useful scoring system for predicting cardiovascular morbidity during pregnancy.
- 4 generic risk factors for an adverse cardiovascular event during pregnancy identified in ♀ with pre-existing congenital or acquired heart disease:
  - Cyanosis.
  - NYHA >2.
  - Impaired systemic ventricular function (EF<40%).
  - Previous adverse cardiovascular event.

Table 17.2 Risk of cardiac event during pregnancy for ♀ with pre-existing heart disease

Number of risk factors present pre-pregnancy	Risk of cardiovascular event in pregnancy
0	5%
1	27%
>1	75%

Physiological response to pregnancy

In the absence of published lesion-specific data, risk can be assessed from whether the heart and circulation are likely to be able to generate the cardiovascular changes that occur in response to pregnancy.

- Lesion specific risk—📖 see Table 17.3, p.219.

Fetal risks

- Any maternal risk.
- Recurrence of congenital heart disease—consider referral for genetic counselling.
- Maternal cyanosis—chance of livebirth 12% if maternal SaO_2 <85%.
- Maternal drugs—e.g. warfarin, angiotensin converting enzyme inhibitors (ACEIs), antiarrhythmics.

---

1 Siu SC, Sermer M, Colman JM, *et al.* (2001). Prospective multicenter study of pregnancy outcomes in women with heart disease. *Circulation* **104**, 515–21.

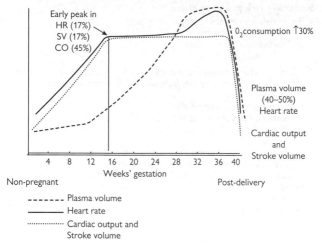

Fig. 17.1 Physiological changes during pregnancy.

Reducing risk pre pregnancy

- Pre-pregnancy surgery or intervention e.g.:
  - Aortic valve replacement for AS; consider valve type.
  - Stent relief of coarctation.
  - Arrhythmia ablation.

NB Consider risk of surgery *vs.* reduction in risk of subsequent pregnancy

- Timing—early pregnancy may be lower risk for some complex conditions.
- Avoid or accept teratogens e.g.:
  - Assess functional capacity off ACEI.
  - Discuss fetal and maternal risk of warfarin *vs.* heparin during pregnancy.
  - Continue to take amiodarone if only antiarrhythmic to control non-ablatable life-threatening arrhythmia → accept fetal risk.
- Treat non cardiac medical conditions e.g. hypertension, diabetes.
- General measures:
  - Take folic acid.
  - Stop smoking.

Pregnancy and delivery

Detailed discussion of the management of specific conditions is beyond the scope of this text.

Antenatal care

All high significant and high risk cases (☐ see Table 17.3) should be referred early to a specialist centre for care by the multidisciplinary high-risk team. The frequency of antenatal visits depends on the individual condition and any complications that arise during the pregnancy.

Delivery

In general, spontaneous, normal vaginal delivery carries the lowest haemo-dynamic maternal risk. Rare cardiac contraindications to vaginal delivery include aortic aneurysm or Marfan with dilated aorta.

A delivery plan including the most appropriate analgesia and the need for invasive monitoring should be documented in the handheld notes. A diagram of the ♀'s circulation should be included if she has complex disease (e.g. Fontan). The ♀ and her team need to be prepared to change the plan if maternal or fetal complications develop at any gestational stage.

Table 17.3 Lesion-specific maternal risk—in the absence of other risk factors

Low risk (mortality <1%)	Significant risk (mortality 1–10%)	High risk/ contraindicated (mortality >10%)
• Unoperated small or mild: • Pulmonary stenosis • Septal defects • Patent arterial duct • Most successfully repaired: • Septal defects • Coarctation • Tetralogy of Fallot • Most regurgitant valve lesions	• Mechanical valve • Systemic RV • Cyanosis, no PHT • Fontan • Marfan	• PHT • Impaired ventricular function (EF <30%) • Aortic aneurysm • Severe L-sided obstruction: • MS • AS

NB Risks are additive e.g: MR with LVEF <30% moves to high-risk category. Mechanical valve with systemic RV moves to high-risk category.

Post-partum

Post-delivery, high-risk cases should be monitored in an HDU setting for 48 hours. The majority of the cardiovascular changes of pregnancy have resolved by the time of a 6–8-week post-delivery cardiac review, but vigilance is needed to detect and manage any long-term deterioration, especially in ventricular function.

Although not supported by prospective or controlled data, there is concern that ventricular function may not return to normal following delivery in some ♀ with heart disease. In particular, the RV (in ccTGA or TGA post-Mustard or Sennning) appears to be particularly vulnerable to the volume-loading effects of pregnancy. It may be hypothesized that such ♀ might benefit from delivery between 36–7 weeks gestation, to avoid the effects of the last few weeks of volume loading on the ventricle.

Endocarditis

Endocarditis prophylaxis

Most congenital heart disease patients have a lifelong risk of bacterial endocarditis (Table 18.1) and hence must be educated regarding:
• Symptoms that may indicate endocarditis and when to seek expert advice.
• Dental health, good oral hygiene, regular brushing, flossing, and need for regular dental check-ups—good dental hygiene and a recent dental check up must be ensured prior to valve surgery or catheter interventions involving device placement.
• Risk of endocarditis with body piercing, tattoos.

Complex congenital cardiac patients requiring dental surgery under GA should be admitted to a specialist centre with collaboration between cardiac anaesthetists, cardiac ITU, maxillofacial surgeons, and adult congenital cardiologists.

Antibiotic prophylaxis

• Current recommendations include UK National Institute for Clinical Excellence (NICE) Guidelines 2008, American Heart Association Guidelines 2007, and European Society of Cardiology Guidelines 2004 (📖 see Table 18.2).
• The lack of concordance between the guidelines reflects the lack of high level evidence. Physicians should use their clinical judgement about whether any particular guideline should be followed for each individual.
• Most people with structural congenital heart disease, surgically corrected or palliated surgical conditions remain at risk of endocarditis.
• The importance of good dental hygiene and aseptic technique for procedures remains of utmost importance and should not be allowed to be overshadowed by controversy about antibiotic usage.

UK NICE Guidelines—recommendations 2008

• Antibiotic prophylaxis against infective endocarditis is **not** recommended for any patient (Recommendation 1.1.3) for:
  • Dental procedures.
  • Non-dental procedures at upper/lower GI tract; genitourinary, gynaecological, and obstetric procedures including childbirth; upper and lower respiratory tract.
• Any episodes of infection in people at risk of infective endocarditis should be investigated and treated promptly to reduce the risk of endocarditis developing (Recommendation 1.1.5).
• If a person at risk of infective endocarditis is receiving antimicrobial therapy because they are undergoing a GI or GU procedure at a site where there is a suspected infection, the person should receive an antibiotic that covers organisms that cause infective endocarditis (Recommendation 1.1.6).

Table 18.1 Risks of developing infective endocarditis or endarteritis in congenital heart disease

Low risk: lesions with no or low velocity turbulence and no prosthetic material

Unoperated	*Operated*
Anomalous pulmonary venous drainage	Anomalous pulmonary venous drainage
Secundum ASD	Secundum ASD
Ebstein's anomaly	Ebstein's anomaly with repaired native valve
Mild PS	VSD/tetralogy of Fallot without residual lesions
Isolated corrected transposition	PDA
Eisenmenger syndrome without valvar regurgitation	Fontan type procedures
	Arterial switch for transposition without residual lesions

Moderate risk

Unoperated	*Operated*
Systemic atrioventricular valve regurgitation	Residual regurgitation of repaired native aortic or systemic atrioventricular valve
Subaortic stenosis	Non-valved conduits
Moderate–severe PS	
Tetralogy of Fallot	
Double-outlet RV	
Univentricular heart with pulmonary stenosis	
Truncus arteriosus	
Coarctatio	
Restrictive PDA	

High risk

Unoperated	*Operated*
Bicuspid aortic valve	Prosthetic valves
AR 2° to VSD or subaortic stenosis	Aortopulmonary shunts e.g. Gore-Tex®, modified Blalock–Taussig
Restrictive VSD	Valved conduits

American Heart Association Guidelines 2007

Antibiotic prophylaxis recommended for congenital heart disease patients at the highest risk of infective endocarditis:
- Unrepaired CHD, including palliative shunts and conduits.
- Repaired CHD with prosthetic material/device within last 6 months or with residual defect at site of prosthetic material/device.

Antibiotic prophylaxis **recommended** in these patients for:
- All dental procedures involving gingival tissues, oral mucosa.
- Respiratory tract procedures.
- Infected skin and musculoskeletal procedures.

Antibiotic prophylaxis is **not recommended** for GU, obstetric, or GI procedures to prevent endocarditis.

European Society of Cardiology Guidelines 2004

- (New guidelines are awaited.)

Antibiotic prophylaxis is recommended for moderate and high-risk patients (□ see Table 18.1) for the following procedures:
- Dental procedures with gingival/mucosal trauma.
- GU procedures.
- Gynaecological procedures in presence of infection.
- Bronchoscopy.
- Tonsillectomy and adenoidectomy.
- Oesophageal dilatation/sclerotherapy.

Further reading

Horstkotte D, Follath F, Gutschik E, et al. (2004). Guidelines on prevention, diagnosis and treatment of infective endocarditis. Executive summary. The Task Force on Infective Endocarditis of the European Society of Cardiology. Eur Heart J **25**, 267–76.

NICE (2008). NICE Prophylaxis against infective endocarditis Guidelines March 2008.
□ www.nice.org.uk/nicemedia/pdf/CG64NICEguidance.pdf

Wilson W, Taubert KA, Gewitz M, et al. (2007). Prevention of infective endocarditis: guidelines from the American Heart Association: a guideline from the American Heart Association Rheumatic Fever, Endocarditis and Kawasaki Disease Committee, Council on Cardiovascular Disease in the Young, and the Council on Clinical Cardiology, Council on Cardiovascular Surgery and Anaesthesia, and the Quality of Care and Outcomes Research Interdisciplinary Working Group. Circulation 116(15),1736–54.

Table 18.2 Summary of recommendations for antibiotic prophylaxis for prevention of endocarditis in congenital heart disease patients (X = not recommended; ✓ = recommended)

	NICE	AHA	ESC
Dental procedures	X	✓	✓
GU	X	X	✓
GI	X	X	✓
Respiratory	X	✓	✓
Obstetric/gynaecological	X	X	✓
GU/GI with infection	✓	✓	✓

NICE National Institute of Clinical Excellence 2008; AHA American College of Cardiology 2007; ESC European Society of Cardiology 2004.

Lifestyle issues

Exercise

Physical activity at an appropriate level has +ve effects both on physical and mental health and should be encouraged in all patients with congenital heart disease.[1]

Many patients with complex heart disease will limit their own activities because of symptoms, but others need guidance to exercise safely.

Exercise for leisure

Type of activity
- Fig. 19.1 classifies sport by type (dynamic, static) and intensity (low, moderate, high).[2]
- Dynamic exercise (e.g. walking, jogging) :
  - Causes—volume loading, ↑ cardiac output and ↑ O_2 consumption.
  - Activity of choice in patients with CHD.
- Static exercise (e.g. weightlifting):
  - Causes—pressure loads on the heart.
  - Less suitable for most CHD patients.

Factors that increase risk of exercise
- Arrhythmia:
  - Extensive atrial surgery (e.g. Senning/Mustard for TGA).
  - Ventricular incisions at surgery (e.g. early-era Fallot repair).
  - Surgical repair of cardiac lesions late in life.
  - Significant ventricular dysfunction (systemic RV, Fallot with longstanding pulmonary incompetence).
  - Previous Fontan-type surgery.
- Pulmonary vascular resistance—PHT may cause syncope and sudden death during more than low intensive exercise.

Recommendations

Simple lesions without exercise risk factors
If no or minimal residual disease—no restrictions.

Complex lesions with risk factors
- No high dynamic or moderate-to-high static exercise.
- Avoid activities that risk bodily collision if pacemaker, conduit, anticoagulated.
- Avoid activities where syncope may be dangerous if frequent arrhythmia.
- Eisenmenger syndrome and any pulmonary arterial hypertension—avoid any strenuous physical activity because of the risk of syncope and sudden death.

Competitive sport[2]

Pre-participation screening
- Full history (including operation note) and examination.
- ECG, echocardiography (residual disease, ventricular function, estimated pulmonary artery pressure), maximal exercise test.

Recommendations

Unrestricted competitive sport only if no or minimal residual disease

Follow-up

- Complete reassessment every 2nd to 3rd year.
- Look for unexpected deterioration (ventricular function, regurgitation, arrhythmia).

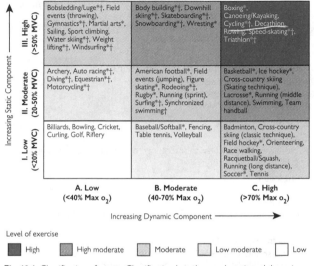

Fig. 19.1 Classification of sports. Classification based on peak static and dynamic components achieved during competition. Higher values may be reached during training. *Danger of bodily collision. †↑ risk if syncope. Reprinted from Mitchell JH, Haskell W, Snell P et al. (2005). Task Force 8: Classification of sport. *J Am Coll Cardiol* 45(8), 1313–75 with permission from Elsevier.

1 Hirth A, Reybrouck T, Bjarnason-Wehrens B, et al. (2006). Recommendations for participation in competitive and leisure sports in patients with congenital heart disease: a consensus document. *Eur J Cardiovasc Prev Rehabil* **13**(3), 293–9.

2 Pelliccia A, Fagard R, Bjornstad HH, et al. (2005). Recommendations for competitive sports participation in athletes with cardiovascular disease: a consensus document from the Study Group of Sports Cardiology of the Working Group of Cardiac Rehabilitation and Exercise Physiology and the Working Group of Myocardial and Pericardial Diseases of the European Society of Cardiology. *Eur Heart J* **26**(14), 1422–45.

Diving

Potential dangers

- Diving reflex:
  - Peripheral vasoconstriction.
  - ↓ HR.
- Immersion in water:
  - Gravitational pooling in legs → fluid shift in to central circulation.
  - ↑ risk of pulmonary oedema.
- Air embolization—↑ risk if previous chest surgery involving opening of pleura, risk of pathological air trapping.
- Decompression illness—↑ risk if R → L shunt.

Cardiovascular requirements for diving

- Normal or near normal exercise capacity.
- Sufficient cardiovascular reserve.
- Absence of R → L shunt.

Specific conditions

Chest surgery

Avoid diving if previous thoracotomy *or* sternotomy involving pleura (e.g. LIMA graft)

Shunt lesions

- Absolute contraindication to diving if ASD or any other lesion that may shunt R-to-L.
- Relative contraindication if PFO or small VSD (diving restrictions may apply).

Obstructive valvar lesions

- Diving should be avoided due to ↑ risk of pulmonary oedema.
- Also contraindicated in hypertrophic cardiomyopathy.

Prosthetic valves

- Avoid diving if mechanical valves—↑ risk of bleeding from cuts and bruises due to anticoagulation.
- Diving safe with tissue valves if no significant degeneration.

Tetralogy of Fallot

- Diving should be avoided if:
  - ↓ exercise capacity.
  - Previous thoracotomy.
  - Residual VSD or significant outflow tract obstruction.
  - Arrhythmia.

Mustard/Senning

Diving contraindicated (abnormal haemodynamic response, risk of arrhythmia and R → L shunt from baffle leak).

Other complex congenital heart disease

Diving contraindicated in all cyanotic heart disease and patients with a Fontan circulation.

High-altitude travel

- Holidays and any exertion at high altitude should be avoided if cyanosis because of ↑ hypoxia.
- Competitive sport at high altitude only if no or minimal residual disease.

Flying

- All commercial aeroplanes equipped with pressure cabins therefore no contraindication to passenger flying with CHD, even if Eisenmenger syndrome[1]. Additional O_2 rarely necessary: temporary fall in SaO_2 well tolerated.
- Precautions for those with limiting disease:
  - Wheelchair/buggy transport within airports to avoid rushing with heavy luggage.
  - Keep well hydrated and avoid alcohol.
  - DVT prophylaxis—keep mobile and wear anti-thrombosis socks for long haul flights.
  - Break long haul flights with >24-hour stopover.
  - Take letter confirming diagnosis, what to do and who to contact in emergency.
  - Appropriate travel insurance.
- Becoming a licensed pilot only possible in unoperated patients with insignificant disease.[2]

1 Broberg CS, Uebing A, Cuomo L, *et al.* (2007). Adult patients with Eisenmenger syndrome report flying safely on commercial airlines. *Heart* **93**(12), 1599–603.

2 Macartney FJ (1984). Flying and congenital heart disease. *Eur Heart J* **5**(Suppl A), 147–54.

Insurance

Patient groups are often the most useful source of information to other patients (e.g. 🖳 www.guch.org.uk)

Travel insurance

Insurance must cover repatriation and emergency medical costs for the congenital cardiac condition. Premiums vary but can be high.

Life insurance

- Life insurance is offered on the basis of long-term survival tables. Such data is lacking for many congenital cardiac conditions, or is based on outdated surgical and medical practice.
- Many with simple lesions are offered insurance at normal or modestly increased rates.
- Those with complex lesions may be offered insurance at very high rates or turned down altogether. Such individuals should seek advice from patient groups or independent brokers before applying.

List of operations for congenital heart disease

List of operations

Arterial switch

- Corrective operation for TGA.
- Great arteries switched over and re-anastamosed to establish VA concordance. Coronaries reimplanted to neo-aorta (formerly pulmonary trunk).
- Restore LV to systemic circulation.
- Brings PAs to lie anterior to the aorta.

Bentall procedure (aortic root replacement)

- Used in aortic root dilatation, aortoannular ectasia, AA aneurysm, and type A dissection that involves the valve.
- AA and AV replaced by a composite graft (i.e. a tube graft with an AV already sewn into it).
- Coronary arteries re-implanted into the side of conduit.

Blalock–Hanlon atrial septectomy (historical)

- Palliative or staging procedure previously used in TGA.
- ASD created via surgical approach (R thoracotomy) without cardiopulmonary bypass.
- Allows mixing of systemic and pulmonary circulations at atrial level to improve arterial saturations.

Blalock–Taussig shunt

- Palliative or staging shunt to increase pulmonary blood flow in PS or pulmonary atresia e.g. tetralogy of Fallot. Often referred to as an arterial shunt or a systemic–pulmonary shunt (to differentiate from venous shunts/connections).
- Classical Blalock–Taussig (historical)—direct anastomosis between subclavian artery and ipsilateral PA.
- Modified Blalock–Taussig—Gore-Tex® tube graft used between subclavian (or innominate) and PAs.
- Can be L or R-sided and be performed via a thoracotomy or midline sternotomy.

Brock procedure (historical)

- Palliative procedure to increase pulmonary blood flow and decrease R-to-L shunt in tetralogy of Fallot.
- Resection of RV infundibular muscle through an RV incision.
- Performed without cardiopulmonary bypass through ether a midline sternotomy or a L anterior throacotomy.

Damus–Kaye–Stansel operation

- Direct anastomosis of the main PA to the aorta to create a single, conjoint arterial outlet to the heart (the main PA is separated from the branch PAs which must be supplied by a shunt or conduit).
- Usually reserved for functionally univentricular circulations to produce an unobstructed systemic outflow in complex aortic and sub-aortic stenosis/hypoplasia.

- Occasionally used in biventricular repair, baffling the VSD through to the neo-aorta and placing an RV–PA conduit.

Double switch operation
- Corrective procedure for ccTGA.
- Arterial and atrial switch.
- Restores the morphological LV to the systemic circulation ('anatomical repair').
- Only possible if the LV is trained preoperatively to work against systemic resistance.

Fontan procedure
- Definitive palliative procedure for functionally univentricular hearts e.g. tricuspid atresia, double inlet LV, hypoplastic L heart.
- Usually preceded by Glenn (cavopulmonary) anastomosis.
- Fontan circulation—IVC and SVC connected directly to PAs. Blood flow though the lungs relies on passive flow (no ventricle) down a venous pressure gradient.
- Pulmonary and systemic circulations are separated (i.e. acyanotic circulation *but* most incorporate a fenestration that allows for a small R–L shunt).
- Classic Fontan—direct anastomosis between RA and PA (called atrio-pulmonary connection, APC).
- TCPC both the IVC and SVC are connected individually into the PAs using a Bidirectional Glenn for the SVC and either:
  - Lateral tunnel TCPC—tunnel created within the RA between IVC and RPA *or*
  - Extra-cardiac Fontan—IVC → PA via extra-cardiac Gore-Tex® conduit.

Glenn shunt
- Palliative or staging shunt to increase pulmonary blood flow (low pressure) in pulmonary atresia or severe stenosis to increase arterial saturations.
- Classic Glenn (historical)—SVC end-to-end anastamosis with the divided RPA (often via R thoracotomy).
- Bi-directional Glenn—end-side anastomosis of divided SVC to the undivided PA (bidirectional implies flow to both lungs). Also called a 'cavopulmonary shunt'.
- Characterized by late development of AV fistulae in the lung(s) supplied by the Glenn.

Kawashima operation (2 meanings)
- 1. Corrective procedure for some types of DORV—intracardiac tunneling of the VSD through to the aorta.
- 2. The name is ALSO used for the use of a Glenn shunt in the setting of azygous continuity of the IVC (usually L isomerism). Thus, the procedure shunts both the SVC and IVC blood to the lungs (effectively a Fontan circulation except that the hepatic veins still drain to the RA).

Konno operation
- Corrective operation for tunnel-type subvalvar AS.
- LVOT enlarged with patch, applied through a R ventriculotomy. May be combined with AV replacement.
- Commonly performed in conjunction with a Ross Procedure ('Ross–Konno').

Mustard procedure and Senning procedure
- Definitive palliative operations for TGA (*atrial* switch procedures). RV still supports systemic circulation and LV the sub-pulmonary circulation.
- *Mustard*—atrial baffle created from pericardium or synthetic material.
- *Senning*—only uses native tissue to create the baffle.
- Baffle directs systemic venous return to LV and pulmonary venous return to RV.

Norwood procedure
- Stage I—palliative (neonatal) operation for hypoplastic L heart syndrome (single ventricle repair) utilizing the RV as the systemic ventricle and creating a systemic shunt to supply the pulmonary circulation.
- Stage II procedure (4–10 months)—bi-directional Glenn to replace systemic shunt.
- Stage III (24–48 months)—completion of Fontan circulation.

Potts shunt (historical)
- Palliative shunt to increase pulmonary blood flow in PS or pulmonary atresia
- DA → LPA direct anastomosis. Difficult to control flow, sometimes caused pulmonary vascular disease.
- Usually performed via L thoracotomy.

PA banding
- Palliative or staging procedure to protect lungs from high flow or pressure.
- Can be used with a view to subsequent corrective surgery—e.g. in neonate with multiple VSDs.
- More commonly used in functionally single ventricle circulations with unrestricted pulmonary blood flow.
- Effectively it is surgically created PS.
- Also used in ccTGA for LV 'training' if considering late double switch.

Rashkind procedure
Staging balloon atrial septostomy in neonates to allow mixing of systemic and pulmonary circulations in TGA prior to definitive surgery

Rastelli procedure
- Corrective operation for TGA + VSD + PS.
- VSD closed with patch that is used connect the LV to the anterior aorta.
- RV → PA conduit.

- Term is frequently incorrectly applied to any procedure involving an RV–PA conduit. It should be reserved for TGA/VSD/PS.
- A Rastelli–Senning operation is a combined atrial switch with Rastelli for ccTGA with a large VSD and PS or pulmonary atresia.

Ross procedure
- Aortic valve replacement using pulmonary autograft.
- Homograft pulmonary valve replacement.

Senning procedure
📖 see Mustard procedure and Senning procedure, p. 234.

Waterston shunt (historical)
- Palliative shunt for severe PS or atresia to increase pulmonary blood flow.
- AA → RPA direct anastomosis. Difficult to control flow, sometimes caused pulmonary vascular disease.
- Often performed via R thoracotomy.

List of syndromes

List of syndromes and their associations

See Table A1.

Table A1 Table of syndromes and their associations

Syndrome	Chromosomal defect	Cardiac defects	Key non-cardiac features	Key facial features
Alagille	20p12 JAGGED gene (AD)	PS, pulmonary artery stenosis	Hypoplasia of hepatic ducts, hepatocellular carcinoma.	Broad forehead, pointed chin, long bulbous nose
Cat eye	22q11 duplication	TAPVD	Renal and bowel anomalies	Coloboma
Cri-du Chat	Deletion 5p	VSD, ASD, PDA, tetralogy of Fallot	Low IQ, growth retardation, high-pitched cry	Round face, flat nose, micrognathia
DiGeorge (CATCH 22)	Deletion 22q11	Tetralogy of Fallot, interrupted aortic arch, truncus arteriosus, DORV	Immunodeficiency, cleft palate low IQ, behavioural and psychiatric disorders	Micrognathia, low-set ears, cleft palate, short philtrum
Down	Trisomy 21	AVSD, VSD, MVP	Low IQ, hypothyroidism, dementia	Upslanting palpebral fissures, tongue protrusion
Edwards	Trisomy 18	VSD, PS and AS	Low IQ, severe growth retardation. Majority die in 1st year.	Small eyes, short nose, micrognathia
Ellis–van Creveld	4p16 (AR)	Common atrium, VSD, ASD, PDA	Thoracic dysplasia, disproportionate dwarfism, 50% die in infancy	Abnormal teeth, sparse hair, 'lip tie'
Holt–Oram	12q2 (AD)	ASD, VSD	Upper limb abnormalities	
Marfan	Fibrillin gene defect (AD)	Aortic root dilation, MVP	Joint disorders, pneumothorax	Lens dislocation, high arch palate
Noonan	12q24 (AD)	PS, HCM	Short stature, bleeding disorders	Triangular face, low hair line, webbed neck

Table A1 Table of syndromes and their associations (*continued*)

Syndrome	Chromo-somal defect	Cardiac defects	Key non-cardiac features	Key facial features
Turner	XO	Bicuspid aortic valve, coarctation, anomalies of systemic and pulmonary venous drainage	Infertile (unless mosaic), osteoporosis, renal anomalies	Similar phenotype to Noonan syndrome
William	Multi-gene deletion 7q11	Supravalvar AS, hypoloastic aorta, PS	Low IQ, hypercalcaemia	Elfin facies—wide mouth, full cheeks, small chin,
Wolf–Hirschhorn	Deletion 4p	ASD, VSD, persistent LSVC	Low IQ, growth retardation. 1/3 die in infancy	'Greek warrior helmet' face

AD autosomal dominant; AR autosomal recessive.

Further reading

Gorlin RJ, Cohen MM, Hennekam RCM (2001). *Syndromes of the Head and Neck*, 4th edn. Oxford University Press: Oxford.

Online Mendelian Inheritance in Man (OMIM™) Y http://www.nslij-genetics.org/search_omim.html

Glossary of terms

Aortography Contrast radiography of aorta to demonstrate abnormalities of the aortic valve, ascending aorta, aortic arch, and descending aorta.

Atresia Congenital or acquired condition in which a valve or artery fails to develop leaving severe stenosis or complete occlusion e.g. pulmonary or tricuspid atresia.

Atrial septal defect Defect in wall between atria.

Baffle Surgically created wall within the atrial mass, for instance in Mustard/Senning or Fontan operations.

Coarctation Narrowing in aorta, typically in the post ductal region but can involve aortic arch.

Conduit Surgical created tube connection, can be valved, between two vascular channels e.g. Fontan extra-cardiac conduit with no valve or valved RV-PA conduit.

Cor triatriatum Membrane within the left atrium.

Cyanosis Arterial saturation <95%

Dacron® Artifical material used to close defects, create conduit and create baffles.

Double outlet right ventricle (DORV) Condition where both great arteries arise from the right ventricle.

Down syndrome Trisomy 21

Ebstein anomaly Abnormality of right heart caused by failure of delamination of tricuspid valve leaflets leading to apical displacement of the valve and atrialisation of the right ventricle.

Erythrocytosis Increase numbers of red blood cells, often as a result of systemic desaturation.

Fontan operation Palliative surgery for univentricular hearts, first performed by Francis Fontan.

Functionally univentricular heart The heart has unequal sized ventricles making a biventricular circulation not possible.

Gadolinium® Contrast agent used in magnetic resonance imaging of the heart.

Gore-Tex® Artifical material used to close defects, create conduit and create baffles.

Hypoplastic left heart syndrome (HLHS) Condition characterised by failure to develop left heart structures, leaving a functionally univentricular heart, with a small left ventricle, small mitral valve, small aorta, and aortic arch

Intra-atrial reentrant tachycardia (IART) Scar related atypical atrial flutter, common in operated congenital heart defects, particularly dangerous post Fontan, Mustard and Senning surgery.

Mustard/Senning procedure (operation) Palliative surgery for simple transposition in which the systemic and pulmonary venous returns are re-directed by means of an intra-atrial baffle to relieve cyanosis. Now superseded by the arterial switch operation.

Patent ductus arteriosus (PDA) Persistence of the fetal arterial duct beyond the neonatal period.

Patent foramen ovale Persistence of the foramen ovale beyond the neonatal period, present in around 25% of the adult population.

Protein losing enteropathy Condition in which there is persistent loss of protein through the GI tract, characterised by low serum albumin and chronic pleural effusions, Ascites and dependent oedema and high fecal alpha1-antitrypsin levels, Carries a poor prognosis.

Pulmonary arteriography Contrast radiography of the pulmonary circulation.

Pulmonary atresia Absence of the pulmonary valve/artery in development, occasionally acquired following severe pulmonary valvar of sub-valvar stenosis.

Pulmonary hypertension Elevation of the mean pulmonary arterial pressure above 25mmHg at rest or 35mmHg on exercise, can be idiopathic or acquired.

Radical repair Term used to describe surgical correction of Tetralogy of Fallot, with resection of the RVOT muscle bundles and patch closure of the VSD ± transannular patch.

Scimitar syndrome Anomalous venous drainage of right lung with anamolous vein passing below the diaphragm to enter into the IVC, with typical 'Scimitar' shadow on CXR. Often associated with sequestered right lower lobe, with arterial supply from descending aorta.

Shone complex (syndrome) Syndrome characterized by multiple left sided obstructive lesions, such as mitral stenosis, sub-valvar and valvar aortic stenosis, hypoplastic aortic arch and Coarctation of the aorta.

Shunt Connection between two blood vessels aimed at increasing blood flow to the distal vessel e.g. Blalock-Taussig Shunt.

Sternotomy Midline incision through the sternum to allow access to the heart and great vessels.

Tetralogy of Fallot Commonest cyanotic heart defect, characterized by anterior superior deviation of the interventricular septum, leading to a VSD, RVOTO, RVH and aortic override.

Thoracotomy Lateral incision in the chest wall to allow access to the pulmonary arteries, aortic arch, subclavian vessels and mitral valve.

Transposition of the great arteries Condition in which ventriculo-arterial discordance is present i.e. the right ventricle leads to the aorta and the left ventricle to the pulmonary artery.

Valvuloplasty Opening of stenosed valve by means of surgical incision or balloon dilatation.

Venesection The removal of one unit of blood to alleviate the symptoms of hyperviscosity in cyanotic heart disease.

Ventricular septal defect (VSD) Defect in the wall separating the two ventricles.

Wood unit Unit of vascular resistance named after the pioneering cardiologist Paul Wood. 1 wood unit is approximately 80 dyne.sec/cm^5

Index